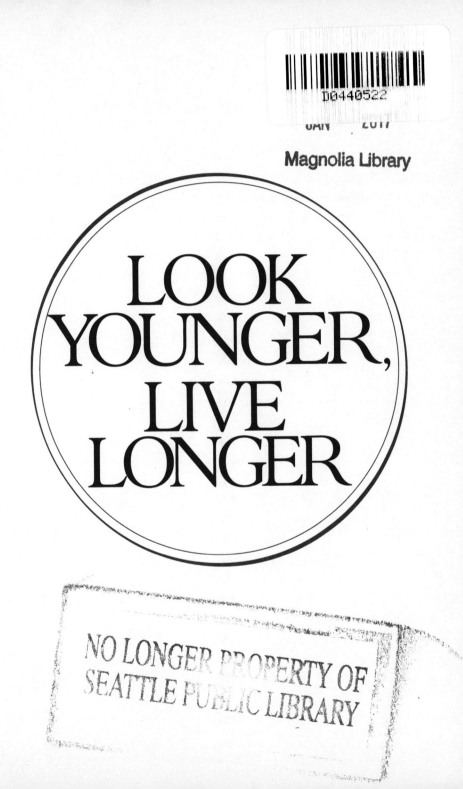

LOOK YOUNGER, LIVE LONGER

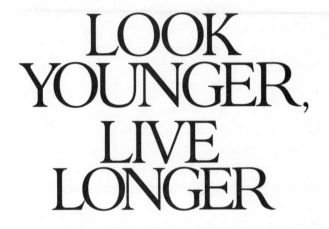

LOOK YOUNGER, LIVE LONGER

FRANCISCO CONTRERAS, MD

SILOAM

Most CHARISMA HOUSE BOOK GROUP products are available at special quantity discounts for bulk purchase for sales promotions, premiums, fund-raising, and educational needs. For details, write Charisma House Book Group, 600 Rinehart Road, Lake Mary, Florida 32746, or telephone (407) 333-0600.

LOOK YOUNGER, LIVE LONGER by Francisco Contreras, MD
Published by Siloam
Charisma Media/Charisma House Book Group
600 Rinehart Road
Lake Mary, Florida 32746
www.charismahouse.com

Visit the author's websites at www.JPCAC.com and www.PediatriciansCareUnit.com.

Cover design by Lisa Rae McClure
Design Director: Justin Evans

Library of Congress Cataloging-in-Publication Data:
Names: Contreras, Francisco, author.
Title: Look younger, live longer / Francisco Contreras, MD.
Other titles: Hope of living long and well
Description: Lake Mary, Florida : Siloam, 2016. | Revision of: Hope of living
   long and well / Francisco Contreras. c2000.
Identifiers: LCCN 2016010456| ISBN 9781629987026 (paperback) | ISBN
   9781629987538 (e-book)
Subjects: LCSH: Longevity. | Health. | BISAC: HEALTH & FITNESS / Healthy
   Living.
Classification: LCC RA776.75 .C663 2016 | DDC 613.2--dc23
LC record available at https://lccn.loc.gov/2016010456

This book was previously published by Siloam as *The Hope of Living Long and Well* ISBN 0-88419-695-X, copyright © 2000.

To my children,

Rose Estela, Marcela, Sandra, Débora,
and Francisco—

may you live long and well

CONTENTS

PART I
THE FOUNTAIN OF YOUTH

PART II
TEN STEPS TO LIVING LONGER,
LOOKING YOUNGER, AND FEELING BETTER

PART III
THERE IS A FOUNTAIN

EXPLORE YOUR POSSIBILITIES

A S A SLENDER nurse closed the delicate lace curtains hanging above her patient's head, sunlight filtered through them, forming a symmetrical pattern on Jeanne Calment's wrinkled face. The nurse set down her tray and whispered in French, "Good morning, madame." Then she touched Jeanne's timeworn hand and walked away to prepare Jeanne's morning bath.

Jeanne's deeply lined eyes opened slightly. Because of the brightness of the sun and the degeneration of her sight due to aging, she could barely see even faint shadows. Turning her head to feel the warm rays that fell on her pillowcase, Jeanne sighed happily as she daydreamed about riding her bicycle around the lovely French countryside. She chuckled softly as her thoughts went to her days in fencing class when each day upon her arrival her teacher would exclaim in French from behind her round mask, "Remarkable!", as she took note of Jeanne's superb physical condition.

And remarkable she was. During the past year, as mentally sharp as always, she had recorded a CD on which she rapped the memories of her long life.

Later that day, August 4, 1997, Jeanne Calment closed her eyes in sleep for the last time. She died gracefully and quietly at the age of 122, the oldest person whose birth date could be authenticated by reliable records. Her birth certificate read

February 21, 1875. She had been born just ten years after President Lincoln's assassination.

Over the years Jeanne Calment had become as notable in Arles, France, as Vincent van Gogh, whom Jeanne had met in her father's art supply store when he visited in 1888. She remembered him as "dirty, badly dressed, and disagreeable."

At the age of eighty-five she had taken up fencing, and she was still riding a bicycle at the age of one hundred. Jeanne Calment credited her longevity to port wine, a diet rich in olive oil, and her sense of humor. "I will die laughing," she had predicted.

Though wheelchair bound, blind, and nearly deaf when she died at a retirement home, she was spirited and mentally sharp until the very end.[1]

LONGEVITY AND HEALTH

As the baby-boomer generation matures through middle age, more and more of us are not only hoping but are also expecting to live longer and more vibrant lives than our parents lived. Powerful scientific breakthroughs promise us the hope of vigor throughout centenarian years. As science begins to unlock the secrets of aging, some of us even hope to defy death altogether. From the beginning of history mankind has pursued the fountain of youth. We have never completely accepted the limitations of time and mortality.

The aging process knows nothing of fairness or equality. Although we all age, we don't age at the same rate. One man is old at thirty, while another dances through his sixties, never feeling or looking a day over forty-five. These disparities in the process of growing older are providing powerful and unique keys for greater understanding. The mysteries of aging are indeed beginning to unravel. With these fascinating breakthroughs in knowledge comes practical insight for beating the clock in our individual lives.

And why shouldn't we use every resource of knowledge available to us to turn back those ticking hands? For regardless of our religious or cultural backgrounds, we all share the love of life and the desire to prolong it as long as possible.

There is no question that the length of one's life is directly connected to one's physical health. According to most physicians, the simplest definition of health is the absence of disease. However, this seems shallow if we compare it with the twenty-four-hundred-year-old definition of Hippocrates, the father of medicine: "Health is the perfect balance between man and his environment." If such a Garden of Eden could exist, what would be the resulting effect on our health and longevity? What if elements of that balance could be restored? Could we all live 120 years, or even longer? Is there real, scientifically verifiable hope for extending our youth? Absolutely yes!

In this book I will examine the roots of our human longing to extend our lives beyond the limitations of time and aging. I will also take an in-depth look at recent medical and scientific breakthroughs that promise the possibility of greatly prolonging our lives. In addition I will investigate with you the genuine possibility of living out your remaining years with enhanced youthfulness, joy, and vitality.

As you explore with me the hope of living long and well, you will discover that it really is possible to live longer, look younger, and feel better!

—FRANCISCO CONTRERAS, MD

PART I

THE FOUNTAIN
OF YOUTH

Chapter 1

IN PURSUIT OF THE FOUNTAIN OF YOUTH

The woods are lovely, dark and deep.
But I have promises to keep,
And miles to go before I sleep,
And miles to go before I sleep.[1]

—ROBERT FROST
"STOPPING BY WOODS ON A SNOWY EVENING"

T HE RUSH OF adrenaline is overwhelming as the airplane door pushes open. Gushing wind rips away breath and speech. Jackets and slacks flap wildly as skydivers charge for their positions. The blood pumping through the heart becomes a throbbing, surreal pulse that seems louder than the wind or airplane engines. In moments that permit no halting movements or second thoughts, each skydiver jumps from the hatch into the nothingness of blue sky.

Does the thought "I'm going to die" occur to them? No. These skydivers jump with an inner conviction—albeit false—that they will live forever. Have you ever wondered why?

THE IMMORTAL BEING WITHIN US

Let's take a moment and carefully examine our mortality and our desire to reach beyond it in pursuit of the fountain of youth.

Some believe that human beings were created to live forever, that we were once eternal beings who eventually encountered death and succumbed to its power. If this is the case, then just where did death begin? Ancient biblical texts state that death started after mankind was created—it was not a part of our original destiny. The Bible also suggests that imprinted into the spirit of each human being is the stamp of eternity.

HUMAN IMMORTALITY?

Adam and Eve enjoyed the cleanest, most unpolluted environment ever in the Garden of Eden. Disease or death did not threaten this perfect balance within their environment. In the Garden of Eden, however, there was one important law: They must refrain from eating the fruit from one single tree. God warned them, "But of the tree of the knowledge of good and evil you shall not eat" (Gen. 2:17, MEV).

We all know the story. This first couple disobeyed and ate the forbidden fruit. But although death was predicted, neither Adam nor Eve immediately fell down dead after eating it. What happened? In my opinion, the instant they sinned by eating the forbidden fruit, the perfect balance was lost. The door of death swung open in both the physical world and the spiritual world.

A dramatic paradigm shift occurred. Originally mankind was meant to live forever. But now we are born, we reproduce ourselves, and then we die. This cycle of life is deeply embedded in our minds after centuries of experience. So why do we still search for the fountain of youth? I believe we still search because deeply ingrained in our genes is the information that we were created to be immortal.

REGENERATION AND IMMORTALITY

An ad for Mercedes-Benz displays a car built in 1955 that, after all these years, shows an odometer reading of a million miles. Its proud owner still enjoys the benefits of his investment. Now, I don't doubt that the Germans produce excellent cars. However, if the car in the ad were a Ford built in Mexico, and if it received the necessary maintenance and replacement of parts, this modest little car would also run indefinitely. By constantly providing the car with new parts, the car would be continually renewed, and it could, in fact, cruise the road forever.

The same renewal process could apply to us as well. Our bodies have a built-in ability to furnish their own spare parts. This ability to replace expired cells is the miracle of life—and it is a trace of the immortality that was lost in the Garden of Eden. If our bodies did not have the capacity to regenerate their tissues, we would not live very long. For example, if our bodies failed to replace red blood cells, we would die in about four months.

Within the extremely complicated organization of our bodies each cell has a different cycle that lasts from hours to years. Some neurons may accompany us for most of our lives, but the rest of our cells are constantly being replaced. For example, the liver we had a few months ago is not the liver we have now, because all the cells within it are new. The same thing is true of all our organs. If this regeneration went on without interruption—if it were not impeded—we would be immortal.

SPECTACULAR LONGEVITY

Immortality was definitely lost at some point after Creation, but some traces of it still remain. And even if total physical immortality is never completely reclaimed, historical records indicate that we should at least be able to enjoy spectacular longevity. Some ancient biblical texts record that characters like Moses, the liberator of the Jewish people, lived 120 years. Even as death approached him, his eyes were not dimmed by blindness, neither had he lost his strength and vigor (Deut. 34:7). Abraham, the father of the Jewish nation, lived 175 years (Gen. 25:7–8). Even more interesting are the records of Abraham's wife Sarah, who, though she lived only 127 years, gave birth at 90 years of age (Gen. 17:17; 21:1–8; 23:1). Amazingly the Bible records that Methuselah, Noah's grandfather, lived for 969 years (Gen. 5:27).

Some critics consider many of the stories in the Bible to be nothing more than myths. But archaeological findings have confirmed the historical veracity of these records over and over again. In addition, it appears that such longevity was not unusual, but rather was the expected life span among the ancient Hebrews.

So what was different about these ancient individuals and their environment that caused them to live so long? According to many experts, the ecosystem before the Flood was amazingly friendly to human life. But we have lost that perfect balance with our world. Today such a perfect environment is difficult to imagine.

Many of us are passively resigned to growing older, getting increasingly weaker and sicker, and then eventually dying. But some prefer to resist it. Poet Dylan Thomas beautifully expressed this resolve to battle aging and death when he said, "Do not go gentle into that good night. Rage, rage against the dying of the light."[2] The human spirit within us does not easily accept defeat. As we move into a new millennium, scientists dream of ways to prolong life.

IMMORTALITY AT THE CELLULAR LEVEL

And the LORD God commanded the man, saying, "Of
every tree of the garden you may freely eat; but of the
tree of the knowledge of good and evil you shall not eat,
for in the day that you eat of it you shall surely die."
—GENESIS 2:16–17

At first glance you might think that the Genesis account places
God in the very difficult position of being found a liar, with
the devil being the one who spoke the truth. For after God's
warning, the devil spoke these words to the first woman: "You
will not surely die. For God knows that in the day you eat of
it your eyes will be opened, and you will be like God, knowing
good and evil" (Gen. 3:4–5).

Since neither Adam nor Eve dropped dead after eating the
fruit from the forbidden tree, at first glance it could seem that
God had lied to them. But since it is impossible for God to lie,
there must be a better explanation. I believe that instead of
Adam and Eve dying on the spot, death replaced immortality
as mankind's new destination.

So, if Adam and Eve didn't physically drop dead, then
where did death take place on that prodigious day? Some of
this judgment occurred at the molecular level, in our human
DNA. DNA is the language of God—God's divine chemical
recipe for the universe.

That day death came in the Garden of Eden, and a recoding
of our DNA took place—our immortality message got scram-
bled. But since the original DNA blueprint wasn't initially
programmed for death, some traces of eternity still remain.
Although our bodies are now encoded to die, some fundamental
place in our DNA simultaneously sends the opposite message as
well. Our DNA also signals us to expect to live forever.

In other words, we were originally coded as eternal beings.

The language that God originally spoke into our cells programmed us for eternity. Therefore, when a skydiver jumps out of an airplane, he is not overwhelmed with thoughts of death. Rather, he is elated by the thrill of life and the defiance of death. The blueprint of God's language deep in the fiber of his being—at a molecular level—signals him that he will never die.

I believe this encoded script is at the root of much of man's search for immortality. The yearning for eternal youth is a theme that can be traced throughout the history of mankind. Every race and nation has dreamed of finding its own fountain of youth.

IN SEARCH OF THE FOUNTAIN OF YOUTH

> Here lie the bones of a lion, mightier in deeds than in name.

These are the parting words written by friends on the epitaph that immortalized the great explorer, warrior, and conqueror whose name in Spanish means "lion." But as I read these poetic lines in a cathedral in San Juan, Puerto Rico, I realized that most of us do not remember the deeds that made him mighty, just the pursuit that made him famous. Juan Ponce de Leon will be eternally linked to the tireless and obstinate human pursuit of the fountain of youth.[3]

Ponce de Leon was born in northwestern Spain in 1460. In 1493 he accompanied Christopher Columbus on his second voyage to America. Ponce de Leon established a colony on Puerto Rico in 1508 and was made governor in 1509. In Puerto Rico he heard a legend about an island called Bimini with a spring that restored youth to all who bathed in it. He was seeking the fountain of youth when he discovered Florida.

This lion explorer sailed from Puerto Rico in March 1513 and arrived at the lush, flower-covered peninsula near St. Augustine on Easter Sunday. Therefore he named the place "la Florida" after the Spanish term for Easter Sunday: *Pascua florida*, or "flowery feast."

Ponce de Leon returned to Florida in 1521. During this visit he was wounded in an Indian attack and was taken to Cuba, where he soon died. The great explorer was buried in the cathedral at San Juan, Puerto Rico. Paradoxically he discovered death in his search for eternal youth.[4]

The legend of the fountain of youth wasn't new to Ponce de Leon. The story was told throughout Europe during the Middle Ages. It apparently originated in northern India and was brought to Europe by travelers and merchants as early as the seventh century. Reference to the fountain can be found in early Hindu writings. In the myths of ancient Greece and Rome there was no fountain of youth within reach of the people of earth, but a spring of immortality existed in the spirit world.

In time the fountain of youth became synonymous with the Semitic legend of a river of immortal life that was found in paradise. Alexander the Great was said to have searched for this magical river in India.[5] So the search for the fountain of youth began long before Ponce de Leon, and it certainly didn't stop with his death. It appears that nearly all cultures have traditions of seeking after the fountain of youth, or after immortality.

The Sumerians

The ancient Sumerians, Abraham's ancestors, had their own legend regarding immortality. Interestingly it includes a story of a flood that covered the entire earth. The myth involves a character called Gilgamesh who seeks the secret of immortality. He learns that one mortal man has been granted immortality: Ut-napishtim. This figure was found virtuous enough to be given the divine guidance to save his family and a remnant of all living things by building an ark in the time before the flood.[6]

What is especially interesting is that Terah, Abraham's father, was a Semite who settled in Ur. The story was part of an oral tradition that dates back almost four thousand years.

China

To ensure a long life, the Chinese have a fascinating tradition of grave clothes. Many Chinese create elaborate burial robes during their lifetimes, employing a young, unmarried woman to do the sewing. They believe that young, unmarried women have many years to live and that part of their longevity will be passed into the clothing. The word *longevity* is embroidered all over the deep blue silk gown.

Since the beautiful garment is believed to possess the power of a long life, the owner wears it often, especially at birthdays and festive occasions, to transfer the power of longevity to his or her body.[7]

Other ancient Chinese traditions seem very peculiar. For example, around 200 BC Emperor Wen of the Nanyue kingdom in the now Guangzhou region of China in Canton had his grave very well planned and constructed by a famous architect of the time. The tomb, made of beautiful red sandstone, had seven chambers, including the reception area, a room for the guards, a kitchen with a large pantry, another room for servants, and a chamber for concubines. You may think that these companions took turns to vigil the dead emperor. The actual tradition was not so romantic. The servants and concubines were all sacrificed so they could attend to the emperor's afterlife needs.[8] I visited the site and noticed that the only door to the tomb was locked from the outside. The door mechanism suggested to me that the companions were locked into the tomb alive. The remains of seven servants, one of whom was a child, and four concubines were found in the tomb with the emperor's remains.

Greece

Demeter and her daughter Persephone were ancient Greek goddesses who were related to corn. The Greeks believed that burying seed in the earth so it would spring up to new and higher life compared with human destiny. They hoped that the grave was the beginning of a better and happier existence in some brighter unknown world.[9]

Egypt

In ancient Egypt the death and resurrection of Osiris, the most popular of all Egyptian deities, were celebrated annually with sorrow and joy. The Egyptians created elaborate pyramid texts and opulent rituals to ensure the eternal life of their rulers. Such texts form the oldest body of ancient religious literature surviving today. These ancient texts protest the reality of death with great passion. Again and again the texts declare that the dead person did not die, but lived. "King Teti has not died the death. He has become a glorious one in the horizon" and "Ho! King Unis! Thou didst not depart death, thou living." In the story of the resurrection of Osiris the Egyptians saw a pledge of life for themselves beyond the grave.[10]

Tibet

Tibetan monks claim to have passed down their own kind of fountain of youth. In the remote reaches of the Himalayas monks created exercises that they say reverse aging. These exercises resemble yoga postures.[11]

Mexico

The Aztecs of Mexico, like other Mayan and Mesoamerican peoples, believed that other worlds existed before their own. The Aztecs believed that one of their gods, Quetzalcoatl, visited the land of the dead and brought back bones with which human beings were created. When he took the bones, the spirits of the underworld warned that they could not be kept forever. The bones would have to be brought back. Quetzalcoatl pleaded that the people who would come from the bones must live forever, but then he lied and told the gods of the underworld that the bones would be returned. As Quetzalcoatl fled with the bones, the gods of the underworld realized his intention and pursued him. He stumbled and fell, and the underworld gods nibbled on the bones, which caused them to rot. As a result, aging would then come to people and eventually result in death.[12]

History is filled with stories, theories, and speculations about death and eternal life. However, if we think that only ancient people concocted such elaborate stories, we are mistaken. Comparable myths, stories, and speculations fill the minds and hearts of people in every century.

MODERN ETERNITY MYTHS FROM SPACE

Many of us recall our horror at learning that young, sneaker-clad Californians committed suicide together in anticipation of the arrival of the Hale-Bopp comet.

Few of us understood their motives. It appears that this group was seeking to transcend this life and go beyond into what the ancients would have understood as eternity. Note this interesting line from their statement of purpose: "Looking to us, and desiring to be a part of my Father's Kingdom [a concept connected with outer space], can offer to those with deposits that chance to connect with the Level Above Human, and begin that transition."[13]

Interestingly even these misguided individuals were seeking the eternal. Every culture on earth, even our own, through elaborate stories, myths, and rituals, sought throughout time for a kind of fountain of youth. These are but a few examples of how mankind, in pursuit of the fountain of youth, searched for eternity that I believe was written into their DNA by the very finger of God.

Just as there has always been a search for the fountain, so has the search always had a darker side to it.

Chapter 2

THE DARK SIDE OF THE QUEST

I want to be immortal by not dying.[1]

—WOODY ALLEN

A
S A BROKENHEARTED lover, Mel Gibson's character allows himself to be cryogenically frozen in a top-secret military experiment. Fifty years later two young boys wander into a military warehouse and stumble upon the capsule containing Gibson's frozen body. After opening it up, they run, spooked by Gibson's icy, blue body. He thaws and searches out the boys by means of a name tag on one of their jackets discarded in their hasty flight.

Over the following few days the young, handsome Gibson searches for remnants of his past. But in bouts of spastic pain, his body dramatically ages fifty years in a matter of hours. The movie ends with Gibson's character and his lover, who was thought dead, now both wizened and gray, embracing in love's redemption of fifty lost years.

Well, that's Hollywood—or is it?

CHEATING DEATH

One can't help but wonder if Gibson's character cheated death by becoming cryogenically frozen or if he simply threw away fifty years of life. It all may sound like spooky science fiction, but such procedures are actually being done right now.

Scientific research and discovery are taking mankind into entirely new, completely uncharted waters—with powerful and sometimes dark ramifications.

Cryogenics

For an average fee of $120,000—which can be procured by signing over your hefty life insurance policy—you can purchase a service that will freeze your body at the point of death. You will be held on ice, awaiting some time in the future when a cure for old age, or whatever ailment brought about your demise, has been discovered.[2]

You don't have that much money to maintain a frozen state? No problem! You can obtain the no-frills package for only $28,000! This will cover your yearly maintenance and the cost of frozen suspension. What a deal! This fee doesn't, of course, include the cost of standby teams and other expenses incurred at the time of your death.[3]

One such organization's advertisement states that the competition would simply "let you die" if you couldn't afford its rates.[4] That is a very interesting statement, especially when you consider that cryogenic procedures can only be performed on those who are already dead. I decided to investigate a little further.

When I questioned an organization as to whether it is possible anywhere in the world to be cryonically preserved before death, I received an interesting reply. I was informed that physician-assisted suicide could be performed under very restricted conditions in the state of Oregon and in parts of Australia. However, I was warned that I should check with local jurisdictions since these laws are in a state of flux.

There are allegations that some organizations use a large number of "premedications" intended to reduce deterioration of the body before deep freezing. The implications and legal questions arising from such procedures are staggering—especially since it is illegal to buy or use prescription medications without a doctor's prescription, and doctors cannot prescribe for persons who are legally dead.[5]

The neuro option

Some organizations offer a particularly macabre version of the cryogenic process called the "neuro," or head-only, technique. After perfusion (introducing a solution that allows the body's cells to survive freezing and thawing), the patient's head is surgically cut off and stored in liquid nitrogen. The rest of the body is then cremated. This saves the organization money since much less liquid nitrogen is required to maintain a single head.[6]

Why would someone even consider such a method? Because it is expected that by the time freezing damage becomes reversible, it will also be feasible to regenerate a new body for the head or to transplant the brain into a cloned, brainless genetic twin. Proponents argue that the brain alone contains the memories and personality of the individual and that preserving the entire body is unnecessary.

CLONING AND IMMORTALITY

Russian author Alexander Lazarevich insists that immortality is technically feasible without the addition of any new scientific knowledge. All that is necessary, according to Lazarevich, is for the technology to be developed based on scientific research now in place.[7]

Other generations have failed in their various quests to achieve immortality, suggests Lazarevich, because all past inventors tried to extend the existence of one and the same body without realizing that what really must be saved is not the body itself, but rather the information that the body contains.

Lazarevich suggests an analogy of an old and treasured

phonograph record. You might try to develop material that would cause the LP to last indefinitely. Or, on the other hand, you could record the LP onto a magnetic tape. When the LP becomes old and unusable, you could simply throw it away and record a new LP from the old tape. Presto—Lazarevich's view of eternal life!

A human being could be considered the same person, according to Lazarevich, if genetic information and memories are transferred from an old body to a new one. How is such a thing accomplished? Cloning!

Lazarevich says, "As soon as you redefine the problem as follows—to preserve the information, rather than the storage media, and to preserve it selectively rather than entirely—the solution to the problem of immortality turns out to be quite trivial."[8]

All it takes is producing a "spare" body that does not have a brain. It could be a person who was in an accident, an individual who was born brainless, or a clone. He agrees that mass production of such bodies might pose ethical questions, but he refuses to address such issues. Data could be transmitted to the new body through "biointerface," or the data interface between any artificial device and the nervous system of a human body. But details are somewhat sketchy regarding how this marvel actually works.

This is only stage one of the project. The second stage would be the production of brain modules. Lazarevich suggests the possibility of growing, out of the body, a brain hemisphere. The new hemisphere and the old could be joined together, and the information from the old could eventually be transferred into the new. When the information has been transferred, a second new brain half could be added. Every time your body wears out, you could repeat this procedure. Voilà! Eternal youth! Lazarevich calls this his recipe for immortality.

Lazarevich isn't the only one who believes eternal life is possible: others argue that "through genetic engineering, nanotech, cloning, and other emerging technologies, eternal life may soon be possible."[9] Ray Kurzweil, for example, firmly believes he will be able to live forever. First, however, Kurzweil has to survive long enough for technology to be developed, and he plans on surviving that long by keeping as healthy as possible and taking 150 supplements a day.[10] Kurzweil wrote that "by the early 2020s, we will have the means to program our biology away from disease and aging."[11]

We may laugh at such notions, but the fact is that they're out there—they actually exist, and people believe them. People are seeking immortality. These efforts are called "transhumanism," which is faith that science will provide us with fantastic longevity and even eternal life.

GENETIC RESEARCH—A PANDORA'S BOX

Some of the greatest recent breakthroughs in the scientific arena are in the field of genetics. DNA molecules are giving up life's secrets, but with such knowledge also come many perils.

Unlike infections, genetic diseases cannot be overcome through our natural defenses. In some cases it is possible to control the symptoms through medical intervention by supplying the missing material of the defective gene. We give insulin to type 1 diabetics, clotting factor to hemophiliacs, and growth hormone supplements to certain dwarfs. Such procedures must be repeated again and again. In contrast, replacing a defective gene or correcting for its loss by adding a normal gene has the potential of being a permanent solution.

Genetic research has impacted liver disease, hemophilia, skin cancer, and other cases of genetic deficiency.[12] Such research has made it possible to cure other genetic diseases in mice. And the basic technology, although still imperfect, could easily be applied to humans.

There is no doubt that genetic diseases are being dramatically impacted by gene therapy. In late 1992 antisense gene therapy testing for fourteen lung cancer patients gained approval from a National Institutes of Health committee of experts. Antisense compounds are messengers that inactivate a gene (in the case of disease, a defective gene), shutting off its signal. Manipulating defective genes produced powerful results.

This may sound innocent enough. But a major ethical issue involves genetic changes that are transmitted from a patient to his or her offspring. It is now possible to evaluate an individual's DNA to determine what, if any, genetic diseases he or she carries. Such information could prove disastrous to certain individuals attempting to obtain employment or medical or life insurance. How will we be protected against those who might attempt to invade our genetic privacy?

Genetic engineering

Genetic engineering therapy has the potential of gradually changing the human race in a directed way.[13] Direct manipulation of genes is not even required. Embryo selection is sufficient once desirable forms of a gene are known. DNA can be analyzed at an early stage in the development of an embryo when it has only four or eight cells. Cells from many embryos can be examined quickly, and an embryo with the desired genetic constitution can then be implanted into the mother's uterus. There the baby develops normally, resulting in a child with the desired characteristics.[14] Such embryonic selection has been in place since the early 1990s and primarily has been used to prevent the births of children with debilitating conditions such as cystic fibrosis or Huntington's chorea. However, its use is being expanded to control things such as sex or cosmetic traits.[15]

Superbabies

Genetic research also holds the potential of genetically engineering a family's blood line and even empowering couples to produce genetically engineered superbabies. Such research is reminiscent of the social engineering first conceived by the Nazi scientists of Germany when Hitler attempted to produce a master race of people.

Genetic engineering could be used to remove undesirable ethnic traits from a nation's population. We could even see gene therapy extended from life-threatening problems to cosmetic ones. Do we have any assurance that such a thing will never be attempted again?

SCIENCE AND ETHICS

The only maxim in science is that whatever can be done will be done. The governments of developed countries are trying to regulate genetic research and development. The restrictions seem ethical. Yet history proves Albert Einstein was right. When he was asked about the dangers of the atomic bomb, he said, "Science…brought this danger, but the real problem is in the minds and hearts of man."[16] There has been no technological advance that has brought good only, from the misuse of shoestrings to strangle people to the unutterable destruction caused by the discovery of atomic energy through the atomic bomb.

If you want to believe that only anarchist movements bring about inhumane experimentation like that of the Nazi doctors, just consider the Tuskegee experiment in which American doctors offered "free medical service" under false pretenses to poor, illiterate people just to research and record the natural course of syphilis.

> Beginning in the 1930s, 399 men signed up with the U.S. Public Health Service for free medical care. The service was conducting a study on the effects of syphilis on the human body. The men were never told they had syphilis. They were told they had "bad blood" and were denied access to treatment, even for years after penicillin came into use in 1947. By the time the study was exposed in 1972, 28 men had died of syphilis, 100 others were dead of related complications, at least 40 wives had been infected and 19 children had contracted the disease at birth.[17]

We know about this awful experiment, but how many such experiments have been done, and how many are ongoing that we do not know about?

For that matter, how many carcinogenic chemicals are lacing our soil, food, and clothing? For years the tobacco industry, through its insistence that smoking does not cause cancer and that nicotine is not addictive, convinced government representatives to maintain its gold mine. We must resist these and other atrocities. Europeans are more politically active than the rest of us, where government officials have banned the use of hormone injections in livestock; they have also banned the importation of genetically altered foods.

The benefits of gene research for crime and medical applications offer hope for improving our living environment, from catching the bad guys to curing diseases and prolonging life. But the greater the benefits, the greater the temptation to misuse the technology.

Scientists have already successfully cloned a sheep and a pig, but human cloning is not yet feasible for ethical reasons.

However, if we develop the technology to create clones of brainless human beings for spare parts, there will be a market for them. If parents can provide advantages to their children through genetic engineering, some will choose this path. If insurance companies can save money by not providing coverage to the genetically challenged, they will. Truly, as Einstein said, the problem is in the hearts and minds of men.

THE DARK SIDE

In the aurora of this millennium, modern-day Ponce de Leons are closer than ever to plunging into the magic waters of the fountain of youth. Today's scientific explorers have taken us into the depth of the human organism to decipher the code of creation's blueprint, DNA, to unlock the mysteries of life with the hope of transcending the stronghold of death.

But mankind's quest to extend the borders of human mortality has always had a dark side. Although most of the experiments that you have read about in this chapter are far from common, such attempts to reach beyond the veil of human mortality are being widely and seriously discussed. And the debates will only become more frequent and heated as science enters into new, uncharted realms of discovery.

The following chapters present an overview of some exciting, although much more common, medical and scientific discoveries in pursuit of the fountain of youth.

Chapter 3

HOW LONG CAN WE LIVE?

Then the LORD said, "My Spirit will not contend with humans forever, for they are mortal; their days will be a hundred and twenty years."

—GENESIS 6:3, NIV

I T WAS COLD, bitterly cold. But it was a good cold. "Good, good," said Grama Alicia with her characteristic intonation, punctuating each *good* with a noiseless clap from her beautiful hands as she leaned her torso forward as if she were in a rocking chair.

Aesthetically those hands were not pretty. They were tainted with the marks of life, emaciated from the work of ages, and diminished from the ravages of calcification. Their beauty was in the history those hands had in almost a century of touching. She put them together without impact as if to protect them from breaking. Most likely she had never heard of osteoporosis, but intrinsic wisdom told her to be gentle.

Grama was excited to have all of her family together to share the wonders of Christmas. For many people Christmas is a party. For her it was a celebration of life. Everybody called her Grama, from the storekeeper at the corner grocery store to her pastor. Her sons and daughters and her great-great-grandchildren knew her only as Grama.

During such times of celebration the matriarch would take charge, patiently allowing every individual to come and pay their respects. Her eyes were dim, but she recognized every individual voice in an instant. The deep creases on her face would radiate like rays of the sun with the sound of each new voice. She kept a mental score as the line got shorter and shorter. After fifty-four souls kissed those corrugated cheeks and forehead, she noted that all were accounted for with her signature "good, good" and her rhythmic bow and noiseless clap. My children have adopted this gesture when something wins their approval, which always brings a soothing caress to our spirits as we remember our Grama.

Everything about the evening was "good, good." The food—excellent. The camaraderie—delightful. It was wonderful to tighten family ties loosened by long distances. All five generations huddled together with our wonderful Grama for a treasured family photo.

Like Grama, more and more of us are not only hoping, but we are expecting to live long and fulfilling lives. The promise of living well into our centenarian years is easily within reach. Scientific advances are rapidly overhauling our expectations, and important advances in age-defying procedures hint at cheating the pain and disability associated with aging completely.

THE LONG-LIVED

What about you? Will you enjoy great longevity? According to current statistics, if you live in Japan, your prognosis is very hopeful. The number of Japanese who live into their hundreds continues to rise dramatically.[1] Japanese women took the lion's share of centenarian ribbons, accounting for 87.3 percent of the individuals over 100 years old. Yasutaro Koide is the oldest living man in Japan at 112; the oldest woman in the country is 115.[2]

In 2013 the Japanese average life expectancy at birth was 87 years for women and 80 for men, making them the longest-lived population in the world.[3] Proportionally Japan has the highest number of centenarians of any country.[4]

The United States is also a good place to live to enjoy longevity. In 1992 there were 36,000 persons in the United States who were 100 years old.[5] In 2015 the United States had 71,972 centenarians.[6]

In the United States life expectancy at birth for women is 81 years, compared to 76 years for men.[7] The average life expectancy has risen from an average of 47.3 years in 1900 to 75.3 years in 1990.[8] The entire elderly population is expected to increase dramatically; 20 percent of the US population is expected to be 65 or older by 2030, which will be an increase of 7 percent from 2010.[9]

CALCULATING LIFE EXPECTANCY

In the twentieth century, life expectancy for women increased about thirty years. In Japan, France, and Sweden the average life expectancy for women increased from 50, 62, and 67 years of age, respectively, in 1940 to 82, 81, and 80 years of age, respectively, in 1990.[10]

For most of recorded human history, average life spans were in the range of 25 to 35 years of age. Now they exceed 70 years in the United States. These statistics may appear more dramatic than they actually are, however. The large numbers of infant deaths, which were a grievous fact of life back then, skewed these numbers. The steep decline in infant mortality accounts mostly for the improvement of life expectancy in the modern world. In the United States and Britain today 98.6 percent of babies are expected to live to age 10, and the population at large can expect to live 74.8 years. Today infant mortality is way down, but the vast numbers of abortions performed every day are not factored into the death rate at all. When abortions are factored in, the figures change dramatically.[11]

In addition, calculations of life expectancy at birth are not an accurate measure of how long any particular individual might reasonably expect to live. On its face, life expectancy at birth is very simple. It reports the average age at death and, therefore, the typical life span of everyone who died during a particular time period—usually one year. However, any specific figure likely understates the life expectancy of a majority of individuals.

FACTS FROM THE PAST

The infant mortality rate in ancient times was astonishingly high. Many of those who did survive to age ten could expect to live, on average, to age twenty-six. Only 150 years ago in the United States and Britain 33 percent of children would have died by age ten.

A thousand years ago, on the island of Cyrus, life expectancy at birth was about sixteen years. But those who survived until age ten appeared to live longer, perhaps into their early thirties. Ancient Rome didn't fare any better. A study of 9,998 epitaphs of early Romans yielded an average life expectancy of twenty-two years.

We are blessed to have been born in this era. Even the countries, cultures, and individuals considered less fortunate experience some of the longest average life spans in history.

WHY DO WE LIVE LONGER?

Obviously medical research has played a role in improving infant survivability, but as social organization and civic order prevailed, as technology improved food supply, and as wars became more limited and more sophisticated (relatively few US soldiers died in the Gulf War, for instance), health status also improved. In summary, the people who live the longest today are the ones who maintain stable, free democracies with a prosperous environment in which healthy, robust people are nurtured and educated and where children are protected from disease, violence, and neglect.

Next to democracy, prosperity is the best predictor of life expectancy. Although the United States is one of the richest nations in the world, it falls at the bottom of the zone, with many nations, albeit all rich, having a longer life expectancy. Switzerland places second to Japan. Virtually all the rest of the advanced, industrialized world falls into a narrow life expectancy zone. The longest life spans in history are found throughout the advanced democracies of Western Europe, North America, and Asia. Achieving a seventy-five-year average life span constitutes an important social and cultural achievement found in only a small fraction of modern-day nations.

THE EVER-WIDENING GENDER GAP

Gender is an important factor in longevity that seems simple at first glance but isn't. Throughout Europe, the United States, and the Pacific Rim women outlive men by large margins. In Greece women live five years longer than men; in Japan, seven years, and in the United States, women live five years longer than men. In the former Communist bloc countries, the differences are larger still: eight years in Hungary and a staggering twelve years in the republics of the former Soviet Union.[12]

The differences persist even though in any given community men and women share roughly the same housing, food, medical system, sanitary conditions, and immunization practices. These facts suggest that female longevity may be influenced in some part through genetics.

If such biological secrets could be unraveled, an additional seven years of life for men would be an extraordinary gain. The steady growth in the female advantage began roughly 150 years ago. It may be that through the centuries women evolved as tougher, more resilient organisms capable of withstanding the trauma of childbirth and the additional stresses of primary care for children.

HOW DIFFERENT NATIONS STACK UP

Even larger differences in average life span may be observed among entire nations. Some examples are given in appendix A. Life expectancy today ranges from an all-time worldwide high of eighty-four years in Japan to a low of forty-six years in the African nation of Sierra Leone.[13] However short its life expectancy may seem, though, Sierra Leone still has more than double the average length of life found throughout most of the history of human existence.

The longest-lived nations eat enormously different diets, although all get plenty of calories. The leader of the pack, Japan, has a diet very low in saturated fat and other animal products and low in fat of any kind. The second longest-lived nation, Switzerland, has more animal fat in its diet than virtually any country in the world except Austria, another long-lived nation. Sharing third place is Greece, with a diet based on monounsaturated fat, or olive oil.

This suggests that the longest life spans the world has ever known are compatible with all three major dietary patterns, providing that nutrition is complete, abundant, and widely available.

Although the well-established maximum human life span of 120 to 122 years is a recent observation, this approximate maximum human life span was recognized long before modern times.[14] Ancient civilizations described ages over 100 as the limits of human longevity and based on records set by individuals. There were probably a few centenarians even in the distant past, but people surviving into their 70s and older were considered to be very old.[15] Michelangelo (1475–1564) and Titian (1488–1576) are two well-known examples from the Renaissance who each lived to be about ninety at a time when most people died at much younger ages due to infectious diseases and violence.[16]

The Bible affirms the maximum life span of 120 years when it says, "And the LORD said, My spirit shall not always strive with man, for that he also is flesh: yet his days shall be an hundred and twenty years" (Gen. 6:3, KJV).

If 120 years is the maximum, why don't we expect to live that long?

YOU CAN LIVE LONGER

Our expectation of living much longer is increasing. And many suggest that 120 years is a beginning point, not really a cap.

By implementing current knowledge, each of us could expect to prolong our lives thirty to thirty-five years. If the genetic mechanisms that control aging, which are beginning to reveal their secrets, are completely uncovered, life might even be extended for one hundred, two hundred, or even five hundred years.

Dr. William Regelson of the Medical College of Virginia believes that in light of recent discoveries, we should be able to add thirty healthy years to human life within the next decade. Furthermore, as we learn to control the genes involved in aging, the possibilities for prolonging life seem practically limitless. A philosophical and good friend of mine, Ricardo Zazueta, heard me speak of these probable accomplishments and commented in a perturbed way, "How awful! Imagine the boredom! The horror of living with the same mother-in-law all those years."

We don't know to what extent scientists will be able to reverse the mechanisms of aging and prolong life. The fact of the matter is that investigations of this biological puzzle are ongoing in hundreds of universities in the United States, Europe, and Asia. In California, for example, one scientist has discovered the genes that cause the aging of skin. In Texas a group of researchers discovered a way to make hundreds of cells reproduce themselves indefinitely. Several groups have discovered genes that prolong life and those that shorten it. Others have detected the switches that turn genes on and off. Biologists have been able to double and triple the life of insects and the life of red blood cells in human beings.

So just how long can we expect to live? To better understand the questions scientists are asking, it is important to gain an in-depth understanding of what happens in the human body to cause it to break down, grow old, and eventually die.

GROWING OLDER: THE THIRD AGE

The presence or absence of disease determines the quality of life in the third age, which begins for most of us at age sixty. In this third age we commonly lose approximately 40 percent of the functional capacities we possessed when we were between twenty-five and thirty years old.

The deterioration is primarily physical. For example, bones are decalcified and cartilage is diminished, which causes an individual's stature to be reduced. This, coupled with poor muscle tone, creates problems in motor coordination, agility, and equilibrium. When we experience these changes, it is not uncommon for us to fall down more often and to suffer injuries from those falls.

Our lungs transport less oxygen to the cells as we grow older. The lack of oxygen, among other things, slows the burning of glucose. Since this is vital to the body's production of energy, we tend to have less energy.

In addition, fat also accumulates throughout the entire body during the third age, especially in the arteries in the form of arteriosclerosis, or hardening of the arteries. The consequences of arteriosclerosis are poor circulation and slower transportation of nutrients to the cells. The heart pumps less blood to the brain, producing cerebral dysfunction, impaired mental agility, loss of memory, and senility. These physical changes can also cause psychological consequences such as anxiety and depression.

If you have aged beyond forty years, you have probably noticed disturbing physical signs of degeneration in your body. In your heart and mind you feel exactly the same as you did ten or twenty years ago, but your body, which once ran swiftly with you, has begun to lag behind. Like most of us, you may have wondered what can be done about it.

There are many theories that attempt to explain why we age, and no one theory answers all the questions. The aging process is complex, and to understand it, we must view it from many angles. So let's take a brief look at some of the theories medical scientists have come up with to help begin to answer your questions.

UNVEILING THE SECRETS OF AGING

Thirty years ago researchers discovered that normal human cells grown in a lab divide about seventy times and die. This suggested that aging and death are programmed into the very building blocks of which we are made. If genes determined longevity, researchers thought that the true secret of prolonging life would be found in regulating those genes and others that control the breakdown of the body.

In 1962 the Nobel Prize for Medicine was awarded to John Watson, Francis Crick, and Maurice Wilkins for discovering the structure of DNA, the hereditary-containing substance found in cells. From that point biologists and other scientists began to ask themselves whether the body contained a

biological clock that determines when a human being should
begin to age. Drs. Calvin Harley, Carol Greider, and Bruce
Futcher found a genetic mechanism that functions as a clock.[17]
The ticking of this clock depends on the length of telomeres,
which are long threads carrying important genetic messages
that cause the cells to regenerate.

When a cell divides, it loses from five to twenty pieces of
the telomeres. When all the segments are gone, the message
is interrupted and the cell stops regenerating itself. Therefore
the length of these threads determines how long a cell family
will live.[18]

The shortening of the telomeres in cellular division may
also contribute to the development of diseases such as arteriosclerosis, osteoarthritis, osteoporosis, and diabetes. Scientists
believe that if they could control the disintegration of the telomeres, then aging could be delayed, and these diseases would
be minimized considerably.

Could the disintegrating of telomeres be the punishment
that Adam and Eve received?

Scientists know that a close relationship exists between the
chromosomes and the genes, which are the building blocks of
DNA. To understand this relationship, it is helpful to imagine
a ladder. Each gene represents one rung, and the chromosomes
are the rails. Every living creature's hereditary information is
coded in these amazing genes.

God created the chromosomes to function as a computer
program whose start-up instructions are written in the genes.
When the chromosomes get instructions from the genes, the
program begins to run. Amino acids come together and form
proteins, which in turn combine to form cells. These come
together to form a plant, animal, or human being, according
to the blueprint found in the chromosomes' program. The
same chromosomes and genes determine the traits of each of

their products, depending on the information they may carry. In humans they determine stature, eye color, IQ, temperament, vocational tendencies, and so on. All of the information about our lives is written in our DNA.

We possess a total of forty-six types of chromosomes. Surprisingly Dr. Carl Barrett discovered that chromosome 1 promotes aging. Dr. James Smith and Dr. Olivia Smith found that chromosome 4 does the same. At a California research company called Geron, Dr. Michael West discovered genes that initiate the aging process in skin cells, blood vessels, and the brain.[19]

Some researchers say that those who inherit tendencies toward long life are not really receiving a longevity gene at all. They are really inheriting a predisposition to longevity that comes by not inheriting other damaging genes that shorten their lives through disease, such as a gene for heart disease.

Thus far the only possible candidate for a life-prolonging gene appears to be one found in individuals with unusually high levels of HDL, the "good" cholesterol that helps prevent coronary disease.[20]

Neuron Loss and Aging

Humans, like other creatures of the animal kingdom, are genetically programmed to reproduce after their kind and raise their young until they become independent. Many scientists believe that aging is a genetically programmed process, just like infancy or adolescence. The fact that some people live longer than others seems to confirm that human development, from cradle to grave, is determined by a genetic clock that signals the various stages of the aging process.

At birth a person possesses some 12 billion neurons. Unlike other types of cells, neurons reproduce themselves very slowly. In the course of our lives we lose a large percentage of these neurons. Some researchers theorize that the main cause for aging might be this neuron loss because the brain controls all organs and their functions. The neuron loss causes the brain to produce a hormone that decreases the body's ability to take in oxygen. This lack of oxygen interferes with the synthesis of proteins and cell division.

Opponents of this theory point out that even species lacking a neuron system as complex as ours still age in a way very similar to humans.

CAN CELLS BE IMMORTAL?

At the University of Texas Southwestern Medical Center, Dr. W. Wright and Dr. Shay discovered two genetic patterns, which they called "mortality one" and "mortality two." When mortality one was activated, cells gradually began to age. When mortality two went into action, cells degenerated rapidly and soon died. By deactivating mortality one, scientists could extend a cell's life between 40 percent and 100 percent. Sooner or later mortality two still went into action and the cells began to decay. But when scientists detained mortality two, the cells began to reproduce indefinitely—they became immortal.[21]

Now the task is to discover if this reproduction can be controlled. Our bodies are predetermined by genetic information, and each person develops according to the blueprint in his genes. In this process a sophisticated balance exists between the powerful stage of growth and the regulatory stage that tells the cells to stop growing. If these opposing forces didn't exist in the universe, or in human beings, nature would be a monstrous disaster. Imagine what life would be like if we didn't have the genes that regulated the size of our noses, our feet, or our height. We would be truly horrible-looking creatures.

Genetic research has brought us amazing discoveries like mortality one and mortality two. Unfortunately the benefits of these discoveries still seem beyond our reach. Yet these same experiments have given us some practical benefits that we can use right now to fight disease and improve our quality of life.

GENETIC ENGINEERING: ARE WE PLAYING GOD?

Thanks to genetic research, hormones like insulin, which were once difficult to produce, can now be made very easily. Scientists can "teach" bacteria how to manufacture these products. They transfer the genetic information to the bacteria, and the bacteria begin to produce the hormone cost effectively. Antibiotics, enzymes, and other medicines are being produced in much the same way. Some bacteria are even trained to eat petroleum and clean up oil spills like that of the *Exxon Valdez*.

Yet all these advances have their risks and costs, to say nothing of the danger of toying with the creation process. What happens when we decide to play God? The fact is, the majority of this genetic research is performed in a laboratory. Scientists know that what happens there doesn't necessarily occur in real life. In my opinion, we are still far from most practical applications of genetic research, and therefore far from obtaining immortality through genetics.[22]

RUST NEVER SLEEPS: FREE RADICALS AND AGING

Other scientists have a different perspective of the aging process. According to Dr. Denham Harman, professor emeritus of the University of Nebraska, aging is caused by the process of oxidation. We have all observed how a peeled apple turns brown or how an abandoned car corrodes over time. These are the result of oxidation. Rust is what happens to metals when they oxidize.

Human aging is similar to what happens to apples and metal in the presence of oxygen. All cells must have a source of energy to maintain life, and that source is oxygen. But oxygen is a double-edged sword. It maintains life, but at the same time it can be very destructive. If a person breathed pure oxygen for two days instead of air that contains only 21 percent oxygen, he would die because his lungs would be destroyed.

Dr. Harman's research led him to propose his theory of aging in 1956. His theory suggests that aging is caused by free radical reactions and may be involved in the aging changes associated with disease and the intrinsic aging process. This theory is now widely accepted in the United States and, indeed, the entire world.[23]

What are free radicals?

Free radicals are among the agents most capable of damaging your body. A free radical is a molecule that contains one or more unpaired electrons in the outer orbit. These molecules react easily with biologic structures, in particular polyunsaturated membrane lipids, DNA, and amino acids. Oxygen magnifies this reaction even more, frequently resulting in cell dysfunction or death.[24]

When an oxygen molecule loses an electron, energy is produced. This process destabilizes the molecule, like untying the knot on a balloon, and it flies around. In its wild flight, the freed electron (free radical) seeks to unite with another electron to stabilize itself. The free radical resolves its problem by stealing an electron from another molecule.

This causes a chain reaction resulting in cellular chaos. The molecules strike furiously against each other in an effort to stabilize themselves, further destabilizing other molecules within the cells. Once the process begins, it is difficult to control. It is hard to imagine that such devastation begins in these tiny little molecules that live only a few thousandths of a second.

Yet every chromosome in our body receives some ten thousand free-radical hits daily.

Free radicals can also interrupt other processes in enzymes and cells, such as hormonal regulation and the development of the proteins necessary to regulate nerves, muscles, skin, and hair. The destructive capacity of the free radicals is enormous, especially because they alter genetic codes. A single free radical can damage a million or more molecules.

Free radicals cause many diseases, including arteriosclerosis, Alzheimer's disease, cancer, high blood pressure, schizophrenia, Parkinson's disease, Down's syndrome, memory loss, brain deficiencies, paralysis, cataracts, arthritis, emphysema, and cystic fibrosis. Without a doubt, free radicals sabotage good health and increase aging.[25] Recent research has demonstrated that environmental and nutritional factors, including pollutants, radiation, pesticides, various medications, contaminated water, and deep-fried foods, as well as physical stress, exhibit the ability to produce enormous amounts of free radicals resulting in tissue injury, disease, and aging.[26]

Cellular degeneration is also suspected of causing aging.

EVERY GOOD THING COMES TO AN END: CELLULAR DEGENERATION

Our bodies regenerate by cell division, which is the mechanism by which our cells reproduce themselves. As we advance in years, our cells don't reproduce themselves as easily as they did when we were younger. In addition, each time a cell divides, the risk of error in this process increases. Inevitable errors result in degeneration and diseases that undermine our health.

For example, cells can become cancerous if their genes don't follow exact instructions. When our bodies reconstruct areas where large quantities of dead and defective cells are located, certain cells move in that reproduce very quickly. To keep tumors from forming, tumor-suppressing genes get involved to help ensure that tissues will grow correctly.

From birth to death, this process never stops. Sadly, with the passage of years, this genetic process is damaged by free radicals and other contaminants. As a result, degeneration and disease undermine health, and the door to aging is opened wide.

In addition to battling free radicals, our bodies must also fight off the effects of toxins.

THE ENEMY WITHIN: ACCUMULATED TOXINS

With the passage of time our bodies find it increasingly difficult to eliminate environmental waste, contaminants, and waste materials produced within the body. For example, as cells make complex substances out of simpler ones—a process called metabolism—they produce toxins. The cells (and their organs) deteriorate because these waste products and toxins aren't eliminated. We go through life accumulating the toxins that gradually hinder important functions and cause our bodies to degenerate. The ongoing battle to remove toxins from our bodies can take a toll on our immune systems.

INADEQUATE PROTECTION: IMMUNE SYSTEM BREAKDOWN

Our immune systems are made of about 70 million different antibodies that protect us from internal and external invaders. This remarkable immune system is policed by electromagnetic and chemical processes designed to recognize enemies—waging an endless war against viruses, toxins, and contaminants that attack our bodies.

On occasion these attacks are so aggressive and frequent that our defense mechanisms get overwhelmed. If the chemical, biological, and emotional stresses are too great, our immune system will become so disoriented that it will attack its own cells, resulting in autoimmune disorders such as arthritis, lupus, and diabetes. We usually experience these diseases in old age, but they can occur in earlier stages of life.

Not only does our body battle viruses and bacteria with our immune system, but this powerful machine must also battle the excesses to which we subject it.

A Sweet but Early Death: Deterioration From Sugar

An excess of sugar in the body, especially refined sugar, causes the proteins within the cells to stick to each other, a phenomenon called cross-bonding. With time, this cross-bonding causes hardening of the joints, loss of flexibility of the blood vessels, and fragile bones. Cross-bonding ultimately causes diseases such as diabetes, arteriosclerosis, kidney disease, and pulmonary disease.

Your sweet tooth can bring on symptoms of premature aging, and so can a couch-potato lifestyle.

Use It or Lose It: Sedentary Lifestyles

Exercising too little or even too much can play a role in the aging process. Two hundred years ago nearly everyone exercised all the time because most people survived by the sweat of their brow. Today exercise is viewed by enthusiasts as a recreational activity—and by the rest of us as a form of torture.

Your body is at its physical peak when you are between twenty-five and thirty years old. From then on it begins to decline. That decline is accelerated through inactivity. Aerobics, jogging, walking, and sports activities slow down the process of deterioration by some 20 percent.

Some studies suggest that vigorous exercise reduces the risk of heart attacks and heart disease. Nevertheless, excessive physical activity can also shorten one's life. For example, the life expectancy of professional football players is shorter than that of the average person.

Various studies support the benefits of both vigorous and moderate exercise. (See chapter 9.) You will have to decide how much exercise is good for you as an individual, paying attention to what your own body tells you and the advice of your physician.

Not only does exercise impact aging, but so does nutrition.

YOU BECOME WHAT YOU EAT: NUTRIENT STARVATION AND OBESITY

Can a person's diet accelerate aging? The answer is absolutely yes. Your body functions by depending on a steady supply of nutrients, proteins, and other substances needed to keep going. Although some of the elements are produced internally, most of them are obtained from the food you eat.

In spite of the body's extraordinary capabilities, it is often impossible for it to convert junk food and chemicals into fuel. On the contrary, these poisons promote deterioration and an acceleration of the aging process.

Our bodies can at least moderately handle most of the toxins and poisons that we pump into them under one condition: that we limit the amounts. But they seem least able to handle too much food and too many chemicals and toxins for extended periods of time. Obesity is a major cause for physical degeneration that leads to aging. In addition, very few obese individuals live into the upper range of longevity charts, which may be another reason the Japanese, whose diet causes them to be far slimmer than some of their Western counterparts, outlive the rest of us.

Few argue that nutrition is directly linked to longevity. We truly are what we eat.

The body's biochemical processes are not unlike the building of a house. Imagine that you just finished building the house of your dreams. Then for some reason you are forced to move to a faraway place like Central Africa. You have the blueprints and a list of all the materials, so you merrily resolve to build your house in Africa.

Upon arriving in central Africa, you experience a major setback. No Home Depot! The materials you need are not available, and those you can find are not of the same quality as those manufactured in your own country. This doesn't mean you can't build a house. But it does mean that your replacement house, in spite of the fact that the same blueprint was used, will not equally compare to the original because of the limited supplies and the inferior quality of the materials used.

The same is true for our bodies. Although all our chromosomes and genes bear all the correct codes and information necessary for the building and replacement of cells, if the materials provided to the body are of inferior quality, the body will produce replacement cells of increasingly inferior quality. Physical degeneration is the consequence of eating foods of inferior quality that have been stripped of their necessary nutrients.

In the same way that a house is only as good as the quality of its materials, the body is only as strong as the quality of the nutrients and other construction materials it receives. If a house has a strong foundation, it can resist external disturbances. However, if the quality of the foundation is poor, or if the foundation is poorly laid, the house may fall. So it is that a deficiency of one nutrient can cause illness, and the absence of a single nutrient can cause death.

AGING: THE BIG PICTURE

We have just briefly looked at several theories of aging. Those who agree that one of these theories or another lengthens life also have strong opinions about what shortens our life spans. But it is doubtful that any one of these theories alone holds the entire truth about aging. Aging happens because of a combination of all of these factors.

All of these theories fit into one of two models. I will summarize them in two parts:

1. Growth factors. Undeniably, our bodies are controlled by growth and growth-inhibiting factors. When we are young, our bodies obviously have an abundance of growth factors that permit them to grow rapidly. As the years pass, the balance changes. The growth factors diminish and the growth inhibitors increase. Lost cells are replaced by fewer fresh cells, and the aging process begins.

2. Reconstruction factors. Our bodies require certain resources for the reconstruction of cells. The codes for cellular reconstruction can be in perfect order, but the quality of the cells that are generated depends on the quality of the construction materials, such as amino acids, vitamins, minerals and so forth. These nutrients require the energy from carbohydrates, proteins, and fats. If these elements are lacking, or if there is insufficient energy to power them, the reconstruction process is less than adequate. In this way too the aging process is accelerated.

You Hold the Keys

Most of us want a long, happy, ailment-free life. But too many of us believe that it is obtained by luck or because of special genes. This kind of thinking is all wrong. Like anything else in life, longevity—living long and well—is achieved by doing the things that are good for us and avoiding practices that are harmful. We each must accept the responsibility for our own health and longevity.

Although genetics and chance play a role in how long you can expect to live, the greatest determining factor is you. You can drastically impact the length and quality of your life. And the human body is amazingly forgiving. Even if you have made all the wrong health choices until now, you can still make a great impact by starting today to make better ones.

With a few exceptions, prolonged health is a personal responsibility. It is something we strive for, not something that is given to us. And good health not only pertains to our bodies but also encompasses the emotional and spiritual aspects that are often ignored by physicians.

At this very moment, barring an incident of fate, you have all the power you need to dramatically increase the length of your own life. You hold the keys to your own longevity, and not only to your length of days but also how you will spend those days as well.

Throughout the next section of this book are ten powerful keys—dramatic ways you can extend your own life span. These keys are built on a broad foundation of medical, scientific, and spiritual truth that can lengthen your life thirty, forty, and perhaps even fifty years or more.

The keys to your longevity are in your hands already. But with informed, well-researched information, I trust you will discover new power to open the door to living 122 healthy years!

PART II

TEN STEPS TO LIVING LONGER, LOOKING YOUNGER, AND FEELING BETTER

Chapter 4

LOSE WEIGHT AND LIVE LONGER

*By suppers more have been
killed than Galen ever cured.* [1]

—GEORGE HERBERT, *JACULA PRUDENTUM*

A WHITE-JACKETED SCIENTIST REACHES into a long cage where a scrawny white mouse is feeding on a few bits of carefully prepared food. Its neighbor in the next cage is plump, round, and robust. But the scrawny one, irrespective of its small size, seems more vigorous and active than its chubby neighbor.

You are looking at one of the most powerful breakthroughs in the history of geriatric and DNA research. These cages contain evidence that rocked the scientific world, evidence that holds the possibility of drastically changing how long you can expect to live. Let me explain.

These mice have proven that by drastically reducing the amount of calories we take in, while at the same time maintaining a high-quality level of nutrition, we can add significant years to our lives. As a matter of fact, if we would eat one-third fewer calories than we normally eat, we could actually lengthen our lives by about twenty-four years. Although many hopeful theories and a great deal of promising research are being done on ways to increase longevity, this theory has been absolutely proven. The method is called caloric restriction.

SUPERCHARGING YOUR HEALTH

Eating a very nutritious diet of 30 percent fewer calories can add 30 percent more time to your life span, in addition to supercharging your overall good health. That means that if you expect to live the average of seventy-five years, you can increase that amount to 97.5 years just by eating less—and you can live healthier too!

Does this seem like an exaggeration to you? Let's look at this astonishing research.

POWERFUL BREAKTHROUGH RESEARCH

Experiments in mice have proven that low-calorie diets block the genes that cause cells to grow old. Drastically restricting calories, along with adding a nutrient-rich diet, has been proven to dramatically lengthen the lives of rats and mice. This method is also being studied in monkeys. However, some of this research isn't new at all.

In 1939 C. M. McCay and a team of scientists reported an astonishing relationship between life span and how many calories rats and mice took in.[2] The life span of these rodents was extended by one-third by drastically reducing calories. Back when these experiments were first conducted, the results were seen as nothing more than an interesting curiosity. But eventually this discovery would form the foundation of a modern breakthrough of information about aging—information that may help you to live longer and maintain your youth and vigor throughout your winter years.

AMAZING DISCOVERIES FROM ANIMALS

Dr. Leon Chaitow tells about Dr. Roy L. Walford, a professor of pathology at the University of California at Los Angeles School of Medicine, who discovered that mice fed as much as

50 percent fewer calories lived nearly twice as long as mice on normal diets. You might think that drastically reducing calories would make them weak and sick. Not so! These hungry rodents were actually healthier and stronger.[3]

Obesity will rob years from our lives. Some researchers say that drastically restricting calories doesn't actually lengthen our life span, but rather it allows us to realize our true longevity potential. Some controversy remains over what is and what is not "normal," with some arguing that since the life expectancy of animals in the wild is shorter than that achieved under "ideal" laboratory conditions, what the experiments are achieving is an actual extension of the natural life term.

Another way of looking at it is that when animals experience the very best conditions in the wild (adequate food and no dangers from predators and climatic extremes, for example), this state is even more "natural" than laboratory conditions. Such a perfect habitat could result in the longer life spans that have only been achieved under laboratory conditions.

But isn't it unnatural to alter basic needs such as food? And can what happens in a laboratory ever be thought of as natural? Maybe not. But these amazing results point to ways in which everyday habits might be modified to give us the benefits of longer, healthier lives. It is, after all, hardly natural that we purify our drinking water. But in just this kind of way, modifications to our eating patterns might become the norm, and while seemingly "unnatural," such changes might allow our true longevity potential to emerge.[4]

In other words, we might have the ability to live longer right now, but we cut our lives short because of how much we eat— even though we consider it to be normal. We are an overfed and undernourished society! Scientists are rapidly breaking new ground as they examine this powerful evidence through the penetrating eyes of dynamic new methods of research.

BREAKTHROUGH METHODS

A revolutionary new method to study aging was introduced in a paper by Thomas Prolla and Richard Weindruch of the University of Wisconsin Medical Center and the Veterans Administration Hospital in Madison.

In the new study Prolla and Weindruch used samples of DNA to show a number of genetic changes in the muscle tissue of normally fed and calorie-restricted mice caused by aging. This new method of studying aging is the most important breakthrough in the history of aging research. For the first time scientists can see the effects of thousands of genes in normal mice and compare these effects to those in calorie-restricted mice whose aging has been slowed.[5]

In other words, scientists have discovered a way to look at the genes so closely that they can see what aging does to them. So they are comparing the genes of mice whose calories are restricted to those whose calories aren't reduced.

Prolla and Weindruch have sweepingly changed the field of aging research forever. This method will dramatically impact all future research in this field. When thousands of gerontologists and clinicians begin applying this new methodology to aging, a rapid explosion in our knowledge will occur. We can expect the human aging process to begin giving up even its deepest secrets in the very near future.[6]

Let me describe just how their method works. These scientists have overlaid new technology in DNA research with the caloric reduction techniques discovered in 1939. In doing so, they have developed the ability to research aging at the deepest cellular level to truly understand why some cells age and others do not.

Dr. Prolla said:

We have used the new technology of DNA microarrays to examine the expression level of thousands of genes during the aging process. We did this in mice comparing five- and thirty-month-old mice. We have learned more in the last three months than in the last three years.

The major advantage with DNA chips is that we are looking at basically all known genes, all the genes that have been well characterized. We start the experiment without the assumption that this gene or that gene will change with aging. We just test them all at once and see what the result is. We get a result that is not biased by preconceived notions. I mean, the only starting hypothesis is that there will be some changes with aging. What the changes are, we only find after we do the experiment.[7]

This method allows scientists to see a broader view of what happens during aging at the genetic level. The old method worked like the story of the three blind men who examined an elephant. The one at the trunk thought it looked like a snake; the one at the leg thought it looked more like a tree; the last one at the tusks thought it looked like a spear. These new methods allow the entire picture to be seen all at once.

By seeing into the molecular level in this way, scientists can quickly find out what factors increase aging and which ones slow it. In addition, the impact of aging on a particular organ, such as the skin, can be tested.

This technique is a powerful breakthrough for understanding diseases. But also, and more importantly, it is a way of measuring the aging process. The only way you can actually reverse the aging process is if you truly have a way to measure it. And with this method we finally do.[8]

The use of animals has been an important part of this research effort. Let me explain how.

WITH A LITTLE HELP FROM
OUR ANIMAL FRIENDS

Believe it or not, the health of a rat's body is very similar to that of humans. Sir Robert McCarrison found that the health and well-being of rats follow closely with that of humans when fed on very similar diets. Therefore results from rat studies are expected to parallel closely what happens in humans. In all the major life extension studies, restricting calories plus increasing essential nutrients caused the animals' life spans to increase as much as 40 to 85 percent. And surprisingly, even though the animals were fed far fewer calories, they didn't become tired and lethargic. Life expectancy increased incredibly without any negative effects on vitality or health. Instead, the animals involved usually appeared more content, more alert, and more vital than did other free-feeding animals.[9]

THE IDEAL RESTRICTED DIET

So just what did the rats eat? Many different diets have been used over the years to get these marvelous results, but the rats in this study were fed diets containing adequate amounts of protein and all other nutrients, only with 40 to 70 percent fewer calories than the animals allowed free access to unlimited food.

Dr. Weindruch and Dr. Roy L. Walford, a professor of pathology at the University of California at Los Angeles School of Medicine, warn that an ideal diet for building a large body and maturing quickly is not necessarily an ideal diet for longevity, which seeks to slow down the biological clocks of the animals concerned. So it is important to be aware of such differences, since creating a diet to effect your own longevity would be less than ideal if you desire to build a Mr. Universe body type.

LOOKING INTO STAGES OF GROWTH

Different rats were studied—some adults, some infants, and others in various conditions of health. When the adult rats were fed restricted diets, scientists felt that they most represented what would happen to people. The best results were achieved when dietary restriction was introduced gradually. In one of their early studies researchers fed normally long-lived adult rats and mice an isonutrient diet that provided just 60 percent of the calories of normal rats. Life spans increased between 10 and 20 percent, with some mice surviving an amazing forty-seven months.

Infant rats on calorie-restricted diets did not experience an enormous life span gain. As a matter of fact, the rats that started in middle age or early adulthood realized about 90 percent of the gain of the rats that were started in infancy. In fact, infant rats had problems. Rats started in infancy experienced stunted growth and a delayed onset of puberty. So, starting later in life has much greater benefits without the negative side effects.

Later, disease-prone rats were given calorie-restricted diets. When these normally short-lived animals were fed far fewer calories according to the plan, the levels of ill health were dramatically reduced (autoimmune conditions affecting the kidneys, for example). The calorie-restricted animals also showed increased activity and greatly outlived their contemporaries who were fed normal diets.

Key researchers agree that there is no question that dietary restriction methods work. They lengthen life and reduce disease in species after species of animals that have been tested. As a result, scientists say that there is no reason whatsoever to suppose that these results will not also apply to humans. Strong evidence already exists that says it does.[10]

DO THINNER PEOPLE LIVE LONGER?

These studies of rats and mice are very interesting, and I agree that these animals probably age exactly as humans. But to really know if calorie restriction methods work for people, researchers needed to find human populations to support it.

The search for population groups who live on restricted diets similar to what was given to the animals netted some interesting results. Several population groups around the world have been reputed as being unusually long lived. These groups include the South American people of Vilcabamba, the central European Caucasian peoples, and the Hunza people of the Himalayas. So researchers decided to look more closely at what these people were eating—and particularly how much of it they ate. They found that the diets of these groups were similar in a number of respects, especially in regard to lower calorie amounts.

Individuals in all three of these groups tended to consume about half the number of calories that adults in Europe and the United States consume. Males took in about 1,600 to 1,900 calories per day, as opposed to 3,300 calories for US males of all ages.[11] The low calorie intake of these three groups certainly helps to prove that a link exists between longevity and restricted calories.

PERFECT HUMAN EVIDENCE

A nearly perfect group of people whose diet very closely resembled the calorie-restricted diet was found. They were the people who live on the island of Okinawa. Weindruch and Walford examined this people group in great detail to see how they compared with the studies on animals.[12] The evidence was powerful.

What made the study even better was that Okinawans have kept excellent and accurate legal records of births and deaths since 1872. Researchers could determine exactly how long everyone lived. In addition, the Japanese Ministry of Welfare and Health had been studying the eating habits of different households for many years by randomly choosing them from all around the country. This gave researchers one more source of information to use.

Most interesting is the fact that more Okinawans live beyond their hundredth birthday than do other Japanese people. While Japan as a whole has particularly long-lived citizens compared with the rest of the world, Okinawans outlive the other Japanese by far. For example, out of every one hundred people who die each year from strokes, cancer, and heart disease in Japan, only fifty in Okinawa die.

The people of Okinawa also seem to be particularly resistant to autoimmune diseases. But this is not because of local genetic traits, but rather because these people simply enjoy an overall better level of health. Schoolchildren in Okinawa eat only 62 percent of the calories per day that the rest the Japanese consume: about 1,300 calories a day. This feature of low calories in children very closely matches the early-life dietary restriction models in research animals.

CHINESE EVIDENCE

The evidence from Okinawa is not unique. In 1982 Dr. Z. Ho of the United Nations University, Massachusetts Institute of Technology, shared his research findings on the diet of an amazingly long-lived people from an isolated mountainous region of southern China.[13]

He examined the eating habits of fifty people between the ages of 90 and 104 (with an average age of 94) who ate mostly maize as gruel with vegetables and oil three times a day. The main vegetables in their diet included groundnuts, sweet potatoes, and rice. Even though their food choices were so limited and their calorie intake well below what is considered adequate by Western dietitians, they ate enough protein—about 10 percent of their total food intake, averaging between 0.8 and 1.1 grams of protein per kilogram of body weight—that they displayed no signs of vitamin deficiency.

Another group of people provided an unexpected look at the results of caloric restriction.

BIOSPHERE STUDY WITH PEOPLE

Dr. Roy L. Walford studied the effects of a low-calorie, nutrient-rich diet of the eight-member crew that participated in Biosphere 2, an experiment to determine if people can live in space, from 1991 to 1993. Biosphere is a nonprofit research affiliate of Columbia University. He was a member of the team and served as its physician inside the glass and steel enclosure called Biosphere 2. During two years in the often-ridiculed experiment, the team grew almost all of their own food.

The Biosphere crew ate a diet that duplicated the calorie-restricted diet given to rodents. They lost an average of twenty-one pounds each through a low-fat menu of mainly fruits and vegetables, with small quantities of eggs, fish, pork, chicken, and goat meat. "The nature of the diet duplicated that shown in rodents to lower the incidence of cancer, diabetes and other age-related diseases and to retard aging," Walford said.

The Biosphere 2 experiment suggests that severe calorie restriction in humans is not harmful to health so long as the diet is nutritious.[14]

RESTRICTING CALORIES IMPROVES HEALTH

In addition to living longer, a calorie-restricted diet has other positive benefits. Cutting calories by 30 percent makes both people and animals healthier.

The scientists locked away for two years inside Biosphere 2 found that their restricted diet of nutrient-dense foods improved their cholesterol, white blood cell counts, blood pressure, and glucose during that time.[15] However, these levels went up again after they got out and returned to former eating habits.[16]

ENERGY-BOOSTING EFFECTS

Does drastically reducing your calories make you tired and lethargic? Researchers say absolutely not!

Monkeys on calorie-restricted diets also enjoyed better health. Dr. Richard Weindruch, a leader in calorie restriction in monkeys, says his chimps can live to be forty years old and are just now entering late middle age. He won't know for another ten to twenty years whether hungry monkeys live longer than monkeys allowed to eat what they like. However, the chimps have fewer cases of diabetes, fewer signs of spinal arthritis, and fewer symptoms of vascular disease.

Still, the skinny monkeys are just as active as their fully fed neighbors.

Studies with mice also support the energy-boosting claims of calorie restriction. Those that could eat all they wanted became sedentary, while those that ate less continued to have energy to exercise.[17]

WHY DOES CALORIE RESTRICTION WORK?

All of these studies have proven that calorie restriction works. But why? What happens in the body to increase longevity as we put down our forks?

Protection from the ravages of toxins and stress

It is not known exactly why eating less increases life span, but experts have several theories. Some believe that the process of converting calories to energy builds up toxins in the body, while others believe that dietary restriction reduces the levels of stress caused by oxidation.

There is little doubt that stress in any form takes a heavy toll. It seems that the body's stressful labor of processing calories can exact a cost in years and vitality.

Less free-radical damage

Eating fewer calories reduces the free-radical damage in humans and animals.[18] This overall reduction in cellular injury from free radicals drastically extends the life of mammals.

When we eat more calories, our metabolism increases. Some researchers believe that this increase in metabolism is what causes a dramatic increase in the numbers of free radicals that are released in the body.[19] As we have already seen, free radicals are major contributors to the aging process.

Reduced DNA damage

In addition to reducing damage from free radicals, calorie restriction reduces DNA damage. C. M. McCay and his coworkers believe that taking in fewer calories impacts the rate of normal damage to a person's DNA, which in turn affects aging.[20]

Investigators compared age-related changes in gene activity in mice fed calorie-restricted (75 percent less food energy) diets to those of mice on normal diets. The results were absolutely fantastic. According to the researchers, the low-cal diets completely or partially prevented 84 percent of the major gene changes usually seen by scientists.

Aging is very destructive to genes. Dr. Thomas Prolla said, "At a molecular level, normal aging looks like a state of chronic injury." He and his colleagues have analyzed more genes with regard to aging than all previous researchers.[21]

Reducing daily food amounts lowers cellular injury and boosts our cellular repair mechanisms, resulting in longer, healthier lives.

Turning On a Light

The hours and hours of research into calorie restriction have turned the light on in many ways. Not only do we know for certain that eating less will lengthen our lives, but we are also discovering a raft of other benefits. Listed below are some of the many promises of calorie-restriction research.

Development of drugs

Researchers now hope that it may be possible to create drugs to mimic the effects of undereating so that we all don't have to go hungry to get the health benefits.[22] But how many of us wouldn't be helped by pushing our plates away a little sooner?

This research may also result in breakthrough skin products that will genuinely keep us looking much younger.

Drug therapies for skin and other organs

In an interview with Reuters Health, Dr. Richard Weindruch said these latest findings may help lead to drug therapies that "retard the aging process…on a tissue specific basis." In other words, skin, the heart, and other organs could be treated through calorie restriction.

Calorie restriction research may also impact aging diseases like Alzheimer's.

Understanding diseases linked to aging, such as Alzheimer's

A team at the University of Wisconsin–Madison has been feeding monkeys a low-calorie diet for years to see if a link exists between calorie intake and age-related diseases.[23] Although their findings are still a long way off, a recent infusion of funds will help them expand this study. We may soon be hearing about some significant breakthroughs in Alzheimer's disease, heart disease, and other conditions linked to aging.

Calorie-restriction research is not only benefiting the elderly.

Breakthrough information will prove useful to all of us, no matter what our age.

Cancer research

Amazingly the calorie-restricted mice studied by researchers had less than half the cancer of normally fed mice. The difference was astonishing. The overall incidence of tumors was 78 percent in the control group versus 38 percent in the calorie-restricted group.[24] This suggests that a link exists between overeating and cancer.

MORE BENEFITS FROM BREAKTHROUGH RESEARCH

Breakthrough knowledge about the damage of overfeeding children

Weindruch and Walford reported that dietary life extension methods are more successful in animals that had not been overfed early in life. The animals that did best when they were introduced as adults to dietary restriction patterns of eating were those that matured slowly and had not been overweight early in life. The message for parents is clear: keep the food intake (and types of food) of children optimal without allowing early obesity to appear.[25]

All of this research certainly flies in the face of current eating trends that encourage us to pack loads of empty calories into our children. What we need to do is feed them—and ourselves—fewer, more nutrient-rich calories.

The results of calorie-restriction research are certainly exciting when you realize scientists are actually beginning to control the length of a person's life. The methods of study promise to open vistas of new knowledge and understanding.

An explosion of information to be gathered from study methods

The power of this method of calorie restriction will lead to an unprecedented explosion of new data about the causes and fundamental mechanisms of aging. This method can (and will) be used in primates (including humans) as well as in rodents, which will revolutionize the field of aging research and lead almost certainly to highly potent treatments to slow down and perhaps even reverse aging in humans in the foreseeable future.

But few of us desire to live longer without the benefits of maintaining our youth. Calorie-restriction techniques can address issues of maintaining youthfulness as well.

Staying younger longer

Researchers say that calorie-restricted mice not only live longer, but they also stay younger. These mice stay younger longer as judged by many age-sensitive markers, which include immune system aging, eye lens proteins, liver enzyme activities, and learning and behavior. So not only does eating fewer calories lengthen our lives, but it helps us to look and feel better too![26]

HOW DOES THIS APPLY TO YOU?

You may be thinking, "Well, calorie restriction seems great for rats and monkeys—but what about me? Will calorie restriction help me to live longer? If so, how do I use this method safely?"

James F. Nelson, an associate professor of physiology at the University of Texas Health Science Center in San Antonio, is looking at what biological mechanisms might be at work in calorie restriction. He said the same physical benefits are seen in almost all the animals that have been placed on low-calorie diets: longer lives, less disease, and more energy. In other words, restricting calories will have the same effect on your life.[27]

Dr. Roy L. Walford absolutely agrees. He says that eating fewer calories and a nutrient-rich diet may very well slow aging and promote better health for all of us.

Some researchers caution that the long-term effects of an extremely low-calorie diet aren't known; therefore it shouldn't be undertaken without a doctor's supervision. Weindruch warns anyone attempting a dramatic reduction in calorie intake to do so with caution. He suggests that those "who elect to pursue calorie-restricted diets should work closely with nutrition experts to avoid malnutrition."[28]

Are you thinking about going on a calorie-restricted diet yourself? Knowing how many calories to cut without causing a negative impact on your health is a little tricky. Several variables are involved, such as your size and activity level. However, according to Dr. Walford, even a 10 percent reduction would be beneficial.[29]

Don't drastically cut your own calories unless you are under the care of a doctor. However, you can probably afford to eat much less food than you do. I suggest that you get down to your ideal weight, or even slightly below it, while keeping your nutrient and protein level high. That extra slice of pizza may taste good on this end, but it could take a slice out of your life span and your prolonged good health.

The first key for staying younger, feeling better, and living longer at any age: lose weight!

Chapter 5

EATING FOR LONGEVITY

Here lies cut down like unripe fruit
The wife of Deacon Amos Shute;
She died of drinking too much coffee
Anny Dominy eighteen forty.

—EPITAPH WRITTEN ON GRAVESTONE

HAVE YOU EVER fought to get in line at the seafood bar at Shoney's? Next time you do, look around for a minute at what today's popular approach to nutrition is doing to everyone's bodies. It will open your eyes. Everyone seems to be getting heavier and heavier and has skin that looks increasingly pasty, ashen, and sallow. The way our society understands and thinks about nutrition is taking us to an early grave.

As we examine nutrition in this chapter, I want you to consider carefully how you think about food and why you eat what you eat. It seems that we all are drifting along in a sea of unhealthy thinking, or lack of thinking, about nutrition and the purpose of food. As you become better educated about nutrition and what it actually does for your body, I hope you will determine to make a fresh commitment to an entirely new way of approaching food and your health.

A visitor arriving at the Oasis of Hope Hospital in Tijuana can enter the dining area on any day of the week and find attractive arrangements of fresh, organically grown vegetables on trays and platters. Our hospital's commitment to organically grown food is part of our holistic approach to cancer treatment. However, eating a diet with plenty of fresh, organically grown fruits and vegetables has another powerful benefit. This diet will lengthen your life and help to keep you looking and feeling younger! Nutrition has been medically proven to be a powerfully effective means of increasing longevity.

If we nourish ourselves adequately, we could prolong our lives by thirty to thirty-five years. Dr. William Regelson of the Medical College of Virginia says that in light of recent nutritional and neuroendocrine discoveries, we should be able to add thirty healthy years to human life within the next decade.[1]

Where is the proof? The Japanese are the longest-lived population in the world. According to Shigeo Takahashi of the National Institute of Population and Social Security, the Japanese owe their surprising longevity to their nutritious, natural diet of fresh fruits, fresh and lightly cooked vegetables, complex carbohydrates, low fats, and very little red meat.[2]

EATING TO LIVE LONGER

If you are like most Americans, and Mexicans as well, you pack your plate with piles of processed carbohydrates, too much refined sugar, loads of saturated fats, and pounds of heavy red meats. Such dietary habits are cutting short our life span. Looking to the Japanese would help us Westerners.

A diet of fresh fruit, vegetables, complex carbohydrates, and healthy proteins will extend your life in two ways.

1. Since poor nutrition and unhealthy dietary factors contribute to disease, changing the way you eat can save you from a premature death.

2. Supporting your immune system with a healthy diet will actually lengthen your expected life span. In addition to living longer, you will actually look younger and feel better too!

Heart disease caused by our poor eating habits is taking a huge toll. According to the National Center for Health Statistics, if cardiovascular diseases were eliminated, the average life span would increase by almost ten years.

Research and epidemiological findings prove that heart disease, hypertension, and cancer of the breast, prostate, pancreas, ovaries, endometrium, and colon are directly linked to poor nutritional habits. What's more, these diseases account for about 60 percent of all premature deaths. If you want to live longer, feel better, and look younger, change the way you eat!

THE SECRET OF
BALANCED NUTRITION

Some people will tell you that all the hoopla about nutrition is overblown—it doesn't really matter what you eat. If you eat regular meals with bread, a few vegetables or sauces and meat, your body will get all it needs. Not true! I'll explain why.

Your computer is a complex machine, and it needs many things to keep it running: energy through electricity, batteries, software, proper maintenance, and much more. Well, your body is vastly more complex than any man-made machine. In the complex process of keeping your body running smoothly, what you eat supplies what is necessary to keep 100 trillion cells doing the millions of different things they do.

What you may not realize is that your body is so amazing that it can find ways to keep working even without getting what it needs. Over the long run, however, this nutritional lack will take a terrible toll in disease, early death, and premature aging. How long and how well you live tomorrow is directly impacted by how well you are fueling your body today.

MACRONUTRIENTS AND MICRONUTRIENTS

What you eat can be broken down into two groups of nutrients according to how much the body needs to function correctly. Those we need in vast quantities are called macronutrients, or high-volume nutrients. Proteins, carbohydrates, and fats are macronutrients.

When we speak of nutrients, we usually think of carbohydrates, proteins, and fats. Occasionally we think of vitamins, yet it is common knowledge that 80 percent of cellular activity depends on micronutrients, or vitamins and minerals.

A balanced diet provides sufficient quantities of macronutrients and micronutrients, despite the fact that some people think that a balanced diet is drinking a soft drink from one hand and eating a cinnamon roll covered with refined sugar from the other. In reality, nearly all foods and vegetables contain both macronutrients and micronutrients, although in different concentrations.

Phytochemicals constitute an enormous group of nonnutritive substances that are abundant in plants and possess health-protective effects. Nuts, whole grains, fruits, and vegetables contain an abundance of phytochemicals, such as phenolic compounds, terpenoids, pigments, and other natural antioxidants that have been associated with protection from and/or treatment of chronic disease, including heart disease, cancer, diabetes, and hypertension, as well as other medical conditions.[3] For example, a banana is considered to be one of the most perfect foods available because it contains all the nutrients needed by the body in the precise amounts needed.

CALORIES FOR ENERGY AND LONGEVITY

When we drive our cars, what is most important is that they run. We want our cars to have all the power necessary to pass another car in traffic or to merge onto a busy access ramp without faltering. We don't stop to think about engine combustion, compression, and temperature. We are only concerned with the car's ability to move. The same thing is true of our bodies. We want them to run properly. But in order to do so, they must have energy.

The quantity of energy released from different foods is expressed generally as Calories. (Note: Calorie [kilocalorie] is written with capital C because it is the equivalent to 1,000 calories—with a small *c*.) Most of us require about 2,000 calories each day, which are obtained from carbohydrates, proteins, and fats.

Carbohydrates: bursting with energy

Carbohydrates are nutritional marvels that are made up of carbon, hydrogen, and oxygen. They energize the body because they are metabolized easily and quickly. Have you ever drunk a glass of orange juice or eaten a piece of candy and felt a burst of energy? It was the carbohydrate power in the food that produced the energy burst. In addition to energy, the waste products generated from carbohydrates are easily eliminated. Carbohydrates also protect liver tissue by helping in the detoxification process. In the heart, they provide the energy that helps the heart contract. In the brain, carbohydrates supply glucose to help regulate the brain's functions.

The vegetable kingdom is the main supplier of carbohydrates. Ideally we should get 70 percent of our calories from complex carbohydrates. The most important sources of complex carbohydrates are vegetables, fruits, cereals, and whole grains.

Body power with proteins

Our bodies are made up of proteins, the second most abundant substance in the body next to water. Proteins regulate energy production and are extremely important in building your body's tissue. They are also vital in the fight against disease. A single cell contains thousands of enzymes, all of which are proteins. Hemoglobin in the blood is a protein. Certain hormones like insulin, glucagon, prolactin, and growth hormone are also proteins.

Most of us think of animal proteins like beef, pork, poultry, fish, and milk when we hear the word *protein*. However, animal proteins like these are difficult for the body to process and use. The molecules of animal protein are extremely complex. Only a small number of them actually benefit our bodies. The rest remain as harmful waste. During digestion and metabolism our bodies break down proteins into amino acids, but the structure of animal proteins requires infinitely more work to break down than do vegetable proteins. In my opinion, vegetarians generally live longer than meat eaters because a vegetarian diet implies less work for the body.

Proteins found in the plant kingdom are also easier for the body to break down and use. Grains such as wheat, corn, and rice and legumes like beans and lentils are rich in protein. Fruits and vegetables also contain proteins. All of these proteins are much easier for the body to break down and assimilate. They also create less harmful waste that collects in the body until it is removed.

Proteins are formed by amino acids, which are their basic building blocks. Amino acids are amazingly versatile elements that unite to form muscle cells, antibodies, and millions of other things. They are made of two parts: an "amino" side and an "acid" side. This duality is the reason for their biochemical adaptability. Essential amino acids are those that we have to ingest because our bodies cannot produce them. Those that our bodies manufacture naturally are called nonessential amino acids. This is something of a semantic blunder because it gives the impression that they are not as important, which is totally incorrect. The reason we don't have to rely on food to get them is because they are *too* important. God must have felt they were so important that He didn't want to chance their shortage, so He designed the human body to produce them on its own.

One of the best ways to ease the body's workload is to ingest amino acids instead of proteins. You can do this by eating plant sprouts. Plant sprouts contain large quantities of essential amino acids, which makes them complete or perfect foods. You could actually live on nothing but alfalfa sprouts and water alone. Granted, after a few months you might start neighing, but you would most definitely be neighing like a healthy horse!

Fat's bad rap

Carbohydrates are your main source of quick energy, but fats are also extremely important to the proper functioning of your body. Fats represent your concentrated stored energy, and they contain more than twice the energy of carbohydrates. When your body lacks enough carbohydrates to provide your energy, insulin is released into your bloodstream, which mobilizes the energy concentrated in fatty tissues to meet the need. Some fat compounds, such as lipoproteins, help your body to use other nutrients, such as the fat-soluble vitamins A, D, E, and K.

Fats are not water soluble, and their structure is very complex. This is why they are more difficult to digest and assimilate than carbohydrates. Fats are essential to life and health. But unfortunately we eat far too much fat, or we eat the wrong kind. Today's fast-food diet forces our livers to work for hours trying to digest the saturated fats found in foods such as french fries, fried chicken, pork rinds, margarine, shortening, and heavy cream. We should never consume more than two tablespoons of fat each day. This includes the oil or butter used to fry foods and the hidden fats in both processed and natural foods.

Those who live the longest take in no more than 10 percent of their calories from fats. Why not try changing your diet in this way? Before long you will discover that you really don't enjoy a heavy, fatty diet after all.

Saturated fats. In general, saturated fat increases the levels of cholesterol in your blood. The most abundant saturated fatty acid in our diet is palmitic acid. Coconut oil, palm oil, whole milk, whole-milk products, and animal fat (chicken, beef, and pork) are the major sources of saturated fatty acids in the diet.[4] Saturated fats are harmful because your body cannot metabolize or use them completely. What your body cannot break down can create fatty deposits in your arteries, causing arteriosclerosis, cardiovascular diseases, embolism, and brain hemorrhages.[5]

Avoid saturated fats as much as possible!

Trans fats. In addition, a relatively new concept in monounsaturated fats involves the concentration of trans-fatty acids in the diet. Trans-fatty acids are created when oils are hydrogenated, a process that converts them into a semisolid state, such as margarine. The content of trans-fatty acids is very high in vegetable shortening, margarine, and, in decreasing amounts, in animal fat shortening and butter fat.

Diets rich in trans-fatty acids elevate LDL cholesterol (bad cholesterol) and reduce HDL (good cholesterol) levels.[6] So limit foods that are rich in hydrogenated vegetable oils, such as stick margarine, cookies, and french fries.

Healthier fats. Olive and canola oils are the major sources of monounsaturated fatty acids in the diet. Recent studies have shown that monounsaturated fatty acids lower blood cholesterol levels when substituted for saturated fats.[7]

Vegetable oils (except coconut, palm, and palm kernel oils)

are rich sources of polyunsaturated fatty acids. These oils include corn, soybean, safflower, sunflower, canola, cottonseed, and soybean oils.[8] The linoleic acid found in some of these oils actually helps to reduce your blood cholesterol levels.

Dietary polyunsaturated fatty acids are classified as omega-6 and omega-3. Omega-3 fatty acids are abundant in fish, shellfish, and sea mammals, especially in those from cold water. These fatty acids are powerful health-boosting marvels, lowering triglyceride levels, reducing the formation of blood clots, and reducing the risk of coronary heart disease.[9]

Choose these wonderful health-boosting fats whenever you can.

EATING WITH WISDOM

In summary, we ought to get 70 percent of our calories from carbohydrates, 20 percent from proteins, and 10 percent from fats. But to strictly adhere to this is difficult because it requires us to limit our choices at each meal.

At this moment I'm eating a healthy snack that tastes like sawdust, which I have to wash down with mineral water. What I really want is a burrito with beans, refried in lard, and a nice, cold Coke. But to live longer and feel better, I have chosen to leave the well-worn path of old bad habits behind to pursue new ones. I encourage you to join me.

THE USEFULNESS OF ENZYMES

Enzymes are proteins that play a vital role in virtually all functions of every organ system in the body. Life as we know it could not exist without the powerful action of enzymes. Enzymes carry out the chemical changes that take place within the cells. Each enzyme has a specific function in the body that no other enzyme can fulfill. Digestive enzymes are secreted along the gastrointestinal tract to break down foods, enabling the nutrients to be absorbed into the bloodstream. Proteolytic enzymes are used to aid digestion and absorption of proteins contained in foods, and they are anti-inflammatory agents.

Your body gets enzymes from two sources: those it makes and those it ingests. However, only raw or uncooked food contains enzymes. Enzymes are extremely sensitive to heat. Even low to moderate heat destroys most enzymes in food. Therefore when your food is steamed, roasted, broiled, stirred, fried, sautéed, candied, pasteurized, or even cooked in a microwave, all of the enzymes in it are destroyed.

Enzymes in raw foods aid digestion of the food so your body's enzymes won't have to do all of the work. So be careful to eat plenty of foods raw as well as cooked. In addition, you can also take enzyme supplements to help prevent the depletion of your body's vital enzymes.

THE FACTS ABOUT FIBER

Dietary fiber gives you proven and sometimes surprising benefits. For the most part, dietary fiber comes from the cellular, structural components and fibrous and woody tissues of plants. While it is true that fiber is neither digested nor absorbed in the small intestine and therefore does not supply energy, it is digested in the large intestine. Here, some of the products of fiber do enter the body's circulation and significantly reduce the production of cholesterol.

There are two kinds of fiber: insoluble and soluble. Insoluble fiber does not dissolve in water, while soluble fiber forms a highly viscous solution when dissolved in water. Insoluble dietary fiber is found in cellulose and in large quantities of whole grains and brans of wheat, rye, rice and corn. It tends to move quickly through the digestive tract where it increases the volume and softness of intestinal content, helping to protect against colon cancer. As fiber moves through our gastro-intestinal tracts, it drags along with it potentially harmful substances, and so it helps to detoxify our bodies.

Soluble or viscous dietary fiber is found primarily in fruits, dried peas and beans, barley, oats, gums (such as guar, xanthan, locust bean), mucilages (psyllium), and pectins. This category of fiber may lower blood cholesterol and help to control blood sugar in diabetes.

The lack of raw fiber in our diets produces constipation, colonic irritation, appendicitis, hemorrhoids, varicose veins, colon and many other cancers, gallstones, obesity, diabetes, and high blood cholesterol.[10]

Most of the grain products consumed in the United States are highly refined. As a result, most commercial foods lose 99 percent of their fiber. The bran layer, or outer layer, and the germ layer, or inner layer, are separated from the starchy endosperm (middle layer) during milling, which leads to the loss of many nutrients and fiber. However, whole-grain products are available in many places. Therefore look for whole-grain products when making selections, and eat lots of vegetables and fruit with the skins.

You should get at least 25 to 35 grams of fiber each day. It is absolutely essential to your good health. To get plenty of fiber, eat lots of bran, fruit with the skins, and whole grains; also take psyllium and other fiber products.

NUTRITION AND CELLULAR AGING

Our bodies have many different systems that must be continually supported through good nutrition. Without the macronutrients we require, these systems will press on, but they will eventually become depleted and will break down.

The importance of this process to the overall aging of your body is easier to understand when you stop thinking of aging as something that happens to your body as a whole. Think of aging as something that occurs at a cellular level. The cells of your body must continually replenish themselves. When you do not provide your body with the nutritional raw materials necessary to maintain cells and their functions, they begin to wear down and become depleted. Skin that once looked fresh and tight begins to sag and lose its color. Joints that once supported your weight with ease begin to hurt and stiffen. By supporting this incredible natural machine—your body—with the very best materials possible, you can maintain the strength and vigor of your entire body for much longer.

FEATURE FRUITS AND VEGETABLES

When you think about dinner or lunch, do you begin with protein? Do you think, "I'll have chicken tonight?" Do steaks on the grill sound like a good meal to you? What about a ham sandwich for lunch?

Have you ever considered building your meals around vegetables? Why is that so unthinkable to you? Are you among the one-fourth of US citizens who get enough fruits and vegetables daily—at least five servings?

If you divided the US population into fourths, starting with those who eat the fewest fruits and vegetables, compared to those who eat the most, you might be surprised. The one-fourth group that eats the fewest fruits and vegetables has double the cancer rate of the one-fourth that eats the most fruits and vegetables. Researchers blame the lack of nutrients, those found in fruits and vegetables, for these shocking statistics.[11]

In addition, recent studies have shown that when animals received the dietary equivalent of a high fruit and vegetable diet with high antioxidant activity, age-related physical declines were reduced. These included retardation in declines in neuronal and mental functioning such as senile dementia (Alzheimer's disease) and even improvement in motor behavior deficits, such as balance and coordination. Not only did this high fruit and vegetable diet slow down aging, but also it actually reversed it in some animals.[12]

Why organic?

Nutritional doctor Walter J. Crinnon describes a patient who showed up at his office one day. He said the large man, over six feet tall and two hundred pounds, felt so awful that he was certain he was dying.[13]

When Dr. Crinnon checked his blood for pesticides, he was shocked. In a test for eighteen pesticides, this man had nine of them. This man's body was poisoned with half of the toxins for which he was tested. Even more alarming is that seventy thousand chemicals are used every day in this country, but only two hundred fifty can be tested for in humans.

This man even tested positive for DDT, which has been banned in the United States since 1972. How is such a thing possible? Even though DDT was banned in the United States, it has not been banned abroad; therefore it can make its way back into our food supply through imports!

Eating foods tainted with pesticides and other chemicals can tax your body with such a heavy burden that you feel robbed of energy, strength, and youth. Eventually, chemically contaminated food can lead to an early death.

Here is another reason to choose organic: the nutrient levels in organically grown foods are higher. In one study the mineral content of organically grown apples, pears, potatoes, wheat, and sweet corn was compared to commercial varieties. Overall the organic foods showed much higher levels of nutrients and much lower levels of heavy metals.[14]

Here are a few of the nutrients that were found in higher levels in the organic foods:[15]

+ Chromium, a micronutrient whose lack in
  Western diets is associated with the onset of
  adult diabetes and arteriosclerosis, was found
  to be higher in organic foods by an average of
  78 percent.

+ Selenium is one of the antioxidant nutrients
  that protects us from damage by environmental
  chemicals. It also helps protect against cancers
  and heart disease. This mineral was found to be
  an average of 390 percent higher in organic foods.

+ Calcium, needed for strong bones, averaged 63
  percent higher in organic fruits and vegetables.

+ Boron, which has been shown to help prevent
  osteoporosis (along with calcium), averaged 70
  percent more.

+ Lithium, which is used to treat certain types of
  depression, was 188 percent higher.

+ Magnesium, which reduces heart attack deaths,
  keeps muscles from going into spasms, and eases
  the symptoms of PMS, averaged 138 percent more.

Other studies suggest that treating plants with certain pesticides can actually lower the level of vitamins in them. The
nutrients affected were vitamin C, beta-carotene, and the B
vitamins.[16]

Researchers also compared the levels of toxic heavy metals
such as aluminum, cadmium, lead, and mercury found in
organic foods to commercially grown varieties. Aluminum has
been linked to Alzheimer's disease. Its content in organic food
averaged 40 percent less than in commercial foods. Lead tox-
icity can also affect IQ scores. It averaged 29 percent lower in

organic foods. Mercury, which can cause neurological damage, averaged 25 percent lower in organic foods.[17]

But if you cannot afford to purchase organically grown fruits and vegetables, then I strongly suggest that you wash your commercially grown vegetables as thoroughly as possible with water. But consider that what you save will cost you dearly with medical bills.

Visit the Mediterranean

A Mediterranean diet is rich in fresh fruits and vegetables, complex carbohydrates, olive oil, and red wine (or red grapes or grape juice). You can also obtain the same effect through supplementation, as we will discuss later.

There is no doubt that eating a diet rich in fruits and vegetables throughout your life will drastically reduce your risk of early death from cancer and heart disease, and it will increase how long you live. Over the past twenty-five-plus years research has shown that those who eat large amounts of fruits and vegetables actually experience less heart disease, cancer, and even cataracts.[18]

The phytonutrients, antioxidants, and nutrition found in fresh fruits and vegetables will strengthen your heart and keep it healthy. Phytonutrients, such as natural flavonoids and carotenoids found in fresh fruits and vegetables, red wine, tea, chocolate, and vitamin C, vitamin E, and beta-carotene also have wonderful cancer-fighting properties.

The Mediterranean diet

We hear much today about the virtues of the Mediterranean diet, but promoting this way of eating is not a new idea. In 1614 Giacomo Castelvetro, a lone Italian voice in the English wilderness, wrote a book called *A Brief Account of the Fruit, Herbs and Vegetables of Italy*. He was horrified by the huge quantities of meat and sweets consumed by his Anglo-Saxon friends. His book is filled with advice that we living at the beginning of the twenty-first century find startlingly familiar.[19]

The term *Mediterranean diet* refers to dietary patterns found in olive-growing areas of the Mediterranean region where culture integrates the past and the present. Much of what is found there today can be traced to the ancient past.

Different regions in the Mediterranean basin have their own diets, making the Mediterranean diet somewhat varied. But olive oil holds a central position in all of the dietary customs and habits of the Mediterranean.

The traditional Mediterranean diet has a total of eight components:[20]

+ High monounsaturated (olive oil) and low saturated fat

+ Moderate consumption of red wine, almost always during meals

+ High consumption of legumes

+ High consumption of whole grains and cereals, including bread

+ High consumption of fruits

+ High consumption of vegetables

+ Low consumption of meat and meat products

+ Moderate consumption of milk and dairy products

HERE'S TO YOUR LONG LIFE

Red wine is an important component in Mediterranean dietary traditions. It is considered the explanation of the

French paradox that coronary heart disease in France is the lowest among industrial countries, despite the high incidence of risk factors such as smoking, a high-fat diet, and the lack of exercise of its citizens. Longevity among the French is often attributed to wine drinking and its positive effect on the heart. Remember Jeanne Calment, the 122-year-old woman introduced in this book? She believed her daily glass of wine was partly responsible for her wonderful longevity.

Wine drinking has been popular for thousands of years. Solomon, the ancient Hebrew king, in the Song of Solomon, the world's greatest love poem, wrote, "Let him kiss me with the kisses of his mouth: for thy love is better than wine" (Song of Sol. 1:2, KJV). Wine later became a biblical symbol in the times of Jesus Christ. During the miracle at Cana of Galilee, Christ turned water into wine, foretelling of the outpouring of His Spirit through the symbol of wine.

Since the earliest times of human civilization wine seems to have been an important and integral component of the human diet. But lately research has revealed that wine drinking actually has a powerful impact on how long you will live.

Through the 1990s an enormous amount of evidence piled up suggesting that moderate red wine drinkers have less heart disease and suffer fewer fatal heart attacks than those who don't drink at all.[21] But don't get the wrong idea. Heavy drinking has never been beneficial. This same evidence proved that those who drank more than just a small amount each day were negatively impacted.

The equivalent of one to two small drinks per day of any kind of alcohol is associated with decreased health risks compared with nondrinkers, while higher amounts result in an increased risk of heart disease and stroke. These observations have tended to characterize light drinking as protective.

The protection has been demonstrated in various population groups for both sexes and all ages.[22]

Some studies found that red wine not only decreased deaths from heart attacks, but it also decreased deaths from other causes. Researchers reported that moderate wine drinking decreased the incidence of breast cancer.[23]

You may be wondering why this is so. Researchers say that up to two servings (240–280 ml) of red wine a day inhibits oxidation of bad cholesterol, or low-density lipoprotein (LDL), thus helping to prevent atherosclerosis. It also increases antioxidant capacity and plasma levels of good cholesterol, or high-density lipoprotein (HDL).[24]

Red wine, but not white wine, contains abundant polyphenols. These are a complex group of compounds that affect the appearance, taste, and fragrance of red wines. They may come from the fruit's skin and seeds.[25] Polyphenols are extremely powerful antioxidants that effectively intercept free-radical activity. The fermentation of red wine helps to release polyphenols, thus making them more available for your body to absorb them.[26]

The two primary phenol groups that occur in grapes and wine are the flavonoids and the nonflavonoids. The most common flavonoids in wine are "catechins" and "anthocyanins" (red-blue pigments).[27] Researchers believe that these powerful substances are responsible for decreased cancer and increased longevity.

However, if you don't drink an occasional glass of wine, I would not recommend that you start. You might consider having a glass of grape juice with your evening meals or for a refreshing snack between meals. Even if the alcohol in wine is thought to release the powerful benefits of flavonoids, it is still the red grapes that provide these benefits. When you consider the dangers and risks involved with drinking, including alcoholism and the subtle encouragement of drinking to those who might have a weaker will than you do, you may choose to avoid the alcohol and yet still receive the benefits of wine through red grape juice.

Drinking tea on a daily basis has the same effect as an occasional glass of wine.

TEA TIME?

Tea has been a favorite hot drink for more than four thousand years. According to Chinese mythology, in 2737 BC Emperor Shen Nung discovered tea for the first time. The tea plant, *Camellia sinensis,* is an evergreen tree belonging to the *Theaceae* family.[28]

The tradition of tea drinking traveled from China to Japan in about the sixth century. The love of tea rapidly spread worldwide, and tea is cultivated in at least thirty countries. Next to water, tea is the most widely consumed beverage in the world, with a per capita human consumption of approximately 120 milliliters per day.

Although there is only one tea plant, tea is processed in different ways. The main types are green tea, which is made by exposing the leaves to hot steam or heat and then dried; black tea, which is made by complete oxidation (fermentation) of the ground leaves; and oolong tea, which is made by partial oxidation of the leaves. Black tea is more popular in Western countries, but green tea is the favorite in Asian countries such as Japan, China, and India. The oolong tea is consumed in Southeastern China and Taiwan.

Thirty to 50 percent of the extractable solids of green tea leaves are antioxidants, especially catechins and flavonoids. A single cup of green tea usually contains about 200 to 400 milligrams of polyphenols, which act as powerful antioxidants. Green tea extracts displayed stronger antioxidant activity than the other types, mainly due to the higher content of polyphenols.[29]

Studies have shown that tea, and especially green tea, has
the potential to prolong life.[30]

YOU NEED THE NUT EFFECT

Traditionally nuts were treated with caution in most dietary
recommendations because of their high fat content. Indeed,
about 60 percent of the weight and 80 percent of the calories
in most nuts come from fat, but this is largely monounsaturated fats (polyunsaturated in walnuts).

Nuts are also full of dietary fiber, micronutrients (for
example, potassium, magnesium, and copper), plant sterols,
and phytochemicals. They are perhaps the best natural source
of plant protein that is high in arginine, the dietary precursor
of nitric oxide, which is a substance that helps inhibit atherosclerosis and lowers the risk of coronary heart disease.[31]

Studies show that eating nuts frequently may decrease
your risk of coronary heart disease by 35 to 50 percent.[32] The
more nuts you eat, the greater your benefits. In a study called
the Adventist Health Study researchers found the following
results:[33]

+ Your fatal heart attack risk is 1.0 if you consume
  one serving of nuts (between 30 to 50 grams)
  less than one time per month.

+ Your risk decreases to 0.78 if you eat nuts one
  to two times per month.

+ Your fatal heart attack risk decreases even more,
  to 0.5, if you eat nuts three to six times per
  week

+ Finally, your risk is reduced to 0.41 if nut consumption is more than one time a day.

In other words, you can cut your risk of suffering a fatal heart attack nearly in half simply by eating a serving of nuts every day! This powerful data is called the "nut effect," and it provides a proven way to extend your life. What could be easier?

What's more, no matter how the data is divided, the "nut effect" is always seen. Men, women, vegetarians, omnivores, smokers, nonsmokers, hypertensives, nonhypertensives, relatively obese, relatively thin, older, or younger persons who ate large quantities of nuts all had a substantially lower coronary heart disease risk than their counterparts who ate lower quantities of nuts. There are no other foods that have been so consistently associated with a marked reduction in coronary disease risk.

Statistics show that those who eat high quantities of nuts experience an extra 5.6 years of life expectancy free of coronary disease. Nut lovers experience an 18 percent lifetime risk of coronary heart disease compared with 30 percent in those who eat low quantities of nuts.[34] So, don't waste any more time! Include nuts in your diet!

LOVE CHOCOLATE FOREVER

Cocoa was probably discovered first by Europeans on Columbus's fourth voyage to the New World in 1502. Recently researchers discovered that chocolate contains large amounts of the potent antioxidant flavonoid polyphenols. A piece of chocolate weighing 41 grams contains almost as much polyphenols as a standard 140 milliliter serving of red wine.[35]

Research suggests that eating chocolate may reduce the risk of arteriosclerosis, heart attacks, and heart disease, thereby prolonging your life. The flavonoid polyphenols in chocolate inhibit the oxidation of LDL (bad cholesterol), helping to prevent arteriosclerosis.[36]

However, don't renew your subscription to Chocoholic's Unlimited. Too much chocolate is bad for you. A similar case of moderation can be made for both chocolate and red wine: too much is as bad as too little.

PERCOLATE LONGER WITH COFFEE

The caffeine found in coffee is also powerful in the body's war against free-radical attack. Caffeine has significant abilities to protect important biological structures, such as cell membranes, from oxygen free-radicals damage.[37] By using it in moderation, those who drink caffeine can benefit from these cancer-fighting effects.[38]

If you have felt guilty over your love for coffee, go and can the guilt. Enjoying a daily cup can actually be a healthy way to start your day!

WHAT ABOUT FAKE FOODS?

In January 1996 the Food and Drug Administration gave Proctor and Gamble permission to sell snack foods, such as chips fried in Olean (the trademark of Olestra), a fake fat. Olean is a bona fide, proven antinutrient. It blocks the absorption of fat-soluble nutrients, many of which play a major role in the prevention of cancer and a host of other degenerative diseases. This substance could cause the deterioration of our health and increase the number of deaths from heart disease and cancer!

Olean is designed to look and taste like fat, but unlike fat, it cannot be absorbed into the body from the intestinal tract. Consequently if you eat a snack fried in Olean rather than one prepared with oil, your intake of calories should be reduced.

On the surface this seems like a win-win situation. However, fake diet foods do not actually reduce obesity. In fact, these deceivers are tied to weight gain.

A study of nurses' health was carried out at Harvard and other medical centers in the Boston area in the 1980s in which nutrition and health practices of almost one hundred thousand nurses were evaluated. According to the study, eating saccharine was the single most reliable predictor for weight gain.

Today's most popular artificial sweetener is NutraSweet, which is found in many products. Yet in the fifteen years after its appearance, the percentage of Americans considered obese skyrocketed from less than 20 percent to over 30 percent.[39]

Olean runs freely through your gastrointestinal tract unabsorbed and is passed out in the feces. It may cause anal leakage, and as fat passes through the intestines unabsorbed, fat-soluble nutrients attach to it and are carried out also. Among these fat-soluble nutrients that are lost are beta-carotene and other carotenoids. Studies reveal that blood levels of the carotenoids may be reduced by up to 40 percent after eating Olean.[40]

Eat as naturally as possible. Don't fall prey to the seduction of fake foods. They fill your body with toxins and actually deplete it of vital nutrients necessary to feel better, look better, and live longer.

HOW YOU EAT MATTERS TOO!

The quality and variety of the food we eat is very important. But for macronutrients and micronutrients to be effective, they must be able to get where they are needed. How you eat and digest your food can keep nutrients from getting where they need to go.

Hundreds of obstacles can keep nutrients from strengthening the body. Here are a few:

+ Not chewing food well

+ Stomach irritated by gastritis

+ Absorption problems in the intestines

+ Deficient chemical processes of digestion

- Intestinal flora destroyed by an antibiotic

- Liver in no condition to metabolize your food

- Arteries coated on the inside with cholesterol, thus restricting passage of nutrients to cells

- Cellular membrane not prepared to utilize the nutrients

- Medicines intercepting the nutrients

You must chew your food long enough to break it down completely, giving it enough time to mix with saliva. Saliva contains many enzymes that are absolutely essential to good digestion.

After your food passes through your stomach, the nutrients it carries must be absorbed through the mucous-covered intestinal lining and be transferred to the bloodstream and the liver.

The liver has the amazing task of feeding our cells since it stores glycogen (an important form of stored energy) and vitamins. It also metabolizes carbohydrates, fats, and proteins. From the liver these nutrients are transported to other parts of the body. As we have seen, each type of cells has its own distinct needs. The powerful liver functions like a chef, attending to some 100 trillion finicky customers.

Your body must overcome these complicated obstacles to maintain good health. It is up to you to facilitate this task. Start by taking smaller bites of food, chewing until it is completely broken down, and swallowing smaller amounts. Never wash your food down with your drink. Don't take unnecessary antibiotics, but when you must, eat a cup of plain yogurt or yogurt mixed with fruit to help reestablish your intestinal flora. These simple steps can go a long way to helping your body appropriate the nutrients your food provides.

CONCLUSION

The safest and surest way to impact your own longevity is through nutrition. I trust this chapter has revealed some surprises as well as fresh insights into good nutrition. The most important key to living longer is balance. If you have spent your life eating because you enjoy certain foods with various flavors, don't stop. But never forget that the real value of food is in the quality of fuel it provides to a fantastically intricate natural machine: your body.

Chapter 6

EXTEND YOUR LIFE
WITH VITAMINS

*We could add an extra twelve to eighteen
years to our lives by taking from 3,200 to
12,000 milligrams of vitamin C a day.*

—DR. LINUS PAULING,
TWO-TIME NOBEL LAUREATE

IN MEXICO, ON June 19, 1994, the newspaper *La Jornada*
published the following news: "Twenty-four million Mexicans are below the minimum levels of nutrition," said
Faviano Dominguez, coordinator of the Program for the Promotion of Health of the Mexican Social Security Institute. As
a country of only 95 million citizens at the time, this figure
represented a staggering percentage of the population.

Even if that stat has improved over time, its affects are
long-reaching. When a country's population is nutritionally
deficient, its national spirit becomes stagnated. Prolonged
deficiency of nutrients results in a slowing of growth, productivity, libido, vigor, energy, and appetite. A country of undernourished and obese people is a country without energy.
When your body is deficient of nutrients, the same thing
will happen to you. You will feel chronically tired, weak, and,
generally speaking, just unwell.

People from developed countries often believe that under-
nourishment is rare because we associate it with places with

famines like Biafra, Bangladesh, and Somalia. But many types of malnutrition exist. You can have plenty of food to eat and still be malnourished if you are not getting all the vitamins, minerals, and other micronutrients your body requires to function properly.

Giving your body the right micronutrients is like a master chef who is given a gourmet assignment. If he is given sufficient ingredients to cook the meal, it is possible for him to cook it. But if he can only count on inferior ingredients, his meal will be inferior. So it is with your body. When you provide the micronutrients your body needs, it will glow with energy, vitality, and health. But when your body must struggle to maintain daily function without vital basic vitamins, minerals, and other nutrients, you can become increasingly weak. This path leads to disease and ultimately to an early, untimely death. It is a proven fact that providing your body with essential micronutrients will increase your vitality, improve your health, and lengthen your life span.

Whatever the cause of malnutrition in the body, doctors tend to forget that sickness is often closely related to it. Sadly enough, thousands of people die every day because they don't have enough food to eat. But even more shocking is that thousands die of malnutrition with their food pantries stocked full of food. These malnourished individuals are filling their bodies with Twinkies, Ho Hos, potato chips, sodas, and white bread—expensive, nutritionally empty foods. In the United States 70 percent of all deaths are linked in some way to eating too much fat, sugar, and salt.[1]

Most of those whose bodies are beginning to fight the battle of aging suffer from deficiencies of vitamin A, vitamin B_{12}, vitamin C, calcium, and iron. The US population in general suffers from deficiencies in zinc, folic acid, vitamin C, vitamin B_6, copper, calcium, and iron.

The body's metabolism is a complex system. We cannot expect that by supplying our bodies with a few chemicals, natural or synthetic, we will instantly attain maximum health and performance. Most often a broad spectrum of substances is needed. When you are young, natural, wholesome food can usually supply most of what you need for energy and health and thereby provide successful nutrition. However, as you age, or in stressful situations such as those provoked by the environment, disease, or extreme conditions such as exercise, eating normal food might not be enough. At the metabolic level aging looks as ravaging to a person's cells as a disease. In these situations supplements can help.

Let's take a closer look at micronutrients and how they can provide a buffer against the cellular war your body must fight against aging.

THE POWER OF MICRONUTRIENTS

Not getting enough nutrients can bring on disease, and the lack of a single nutrient can even cause death. In 1750 James Lind was the first to scientifically demonstrate that foods not only have the function of satisfying hunger, but they also contain essential elements that our bodies cannot produce—elements that determine our physical and even our mental health.

Lind also discovered the relationship between the lack of specific nutrients and disease. In 1747 he made the first classical study of mariners who suffered from scurvy. For these men he prescribed specific foods. Those individuals who ate oranges and lemons got well in six days. This discovery saved the lives of countless seafaring men who simply began carrying oranges and lemons onboard, which is why sailors received the nickname "limies." Through this breakthrough discovery Dr. Lind established the link between types of food and health.

Lind published his conclusions in 1753 in a work titled "A Treatise of the Scurvy." Twenty years had to pass before Lind's findings made an international impact. In those days there was neither telephone nor telegraph, and no worldwide medical conventions.

The era of scientific nutrition began 160 years after Lind's discovery. In 1912 Dr. Casimir Funk discovered thiamin (vitamin B$_1$). His discovery helped cure a disease known as beriberi.[2] Still medical science has often resisted nutritional solutions for disease, choosing instead to seek for answers through drug research. However, the impact of vitamins on our bodies should not be underestimated.

GIVE YOUR BODY THE BEST RESOURCES

Have you ever planted a garden or tried to grow a single plant? If so, you have learned that plants need continual care. If you water them and give them good soil and occasional plant food, they will grow and thrive. If you give them even more plant food and all the sunlight and water they need, they will flourish and produce fruit. With optimum care you can increase their hardiness and fruitfulness, and you can significantly impact their longevity.

Your body is really not much different. If you give your body all the vitamins, minerals, and other nutrients it needs, you will end up with a much different body than one that is neglected and poorly cared for—especially in terms of health, energy, hardiness, and longevity.

Providing the very best resources for your body has a dramatic effect. You can see the dramatic impact of nutrients in plants that have a much shorter life span. The impact of a lack of nutrients over time on the human body is even more dramatic, although it may be less obvious at first. An individual whose body is deprived of vital nutrients will probably not notice a great affect for years, unless the deprivation is very severe. This person will contact colds, flu, and other diseases more often. He or she may enter middle age feeling fatigued all the time and generally unwell. Eventually chronic fatigue and serious disease will follow, with the end result being a premature death.

This doesn't have to happen to you. You can choose to provide your body with all it needs for optimal health. Begin learning what micronutrients your body requires. The sooner you begin giving your body everything it needs for peak performance, the better. If you are younger than thirty-five years, you can get all of the micronutrients your body requires by eating a healthy, well-balanced diet and taking a good daily multivitamin/multimineral supplement. If you are older than thirty-five years, be aware that the aging process that has already begun to take place in your body at the cellular level has the same devastating effect on your cells as a ravaging disease. You must begin to counter this effect by becoming very smart regarding your body's micronutrient requirements.

THE SUPER EFFECT OF SUPPLEMENTS

As I see it, it is necessary to consume very high quantities of nutrients to maintain health, especially throughout middle age and beyond. Today many doctors insist that a correctly balanced diet should not demand nutritional supplements. This might have been true two hundred to three hundred years ago before the food industry began to heavily manipulate our food supply. But today nutritional supplements are absolutely essential.

Let's look at some supplements that will prove invaluable to your health and longevity.

VITAMINS AND VITALITY

The word *vitamin* was invented by Casimir Funk while looking for the cause of beriberi. He wanted a term that would distinguish a nutrient that is neither protein, carbohydrate, fat nor mineral.[3]

Vitamins act mainly as coenzymes. They are not building blocks of the body like proteins. They don't produce energy. They are not even basic elements. Vitamins improve metabolism, prevent disease, and help slow down the aging process. Our health problems would be greatly reduced if we would take vitamins in adequate quantities.

Let's take a look at some vitamin supplements that can dramatically lengthen your life.

ADD YEARS WITH VITAMIN C

Vitamin C has been proven to add years to your life, according to Dr. Linus Pauling, two-time Nobel Prize–winning scientist. He strongly believed that he lengthened his own life span by twenty years by taking megadoses of vitamin C.[4]

A large body of evidence is beginning to prove Pauling right. Even low doses of vitamin C can give your life expectancy a real boost. "We've now got the first solid proof that vitamin C can add years to your life," says Morton A. Klein. According to Klein, "Deaths from cardiovascular disease alone dropped by over 40 percent in the male vitamin C takers." Klein and UCLA's James E. Engstrom, PhD, analyzed government dietary intakes of eleven thousand Americans. They found that getting 300 milligrams of vitamin C daily (roughly half in supplements) added six years to a man's life and two years to a woman's life.[5]

According to Engstrom, the remarkable life-prolonging benefits from vitamin C by far outdistance what you can expect from lowering your cholesterol and cutting down on fat. Those who take vitamin C live longer even if they smoke, eat poor diets, and lack exercise.[6]

Epidemiologic evidence and extensive research has shown that vitamin C is a powerful antioxidant.[7] It also helps protect the body from various pollutants, including the toxins caused by cigarette smoke.[8] In addition, vitamin C supplementation has been found to reduce the risk of cerebrovascular disease and dementia.[9]

Dr. Pauling died of cancer at the age of ninety-three. Before he died, he said, "I have to attribute my health at this point largely to my intake of vitamins and minerals." Although he died of cancer, he believed vitamins had delayed the onset of the cancer by about twenty years. He claimed to have had no colds since he began taking high doses of vitamin C in 1965. He started taking a single vitamin pill in 1941. Eventually he ingested 18,000 milligrams of vitamin C daily.

The Nobel Prize winner believed that we could live an extra twelve to eighteen years if we took 3,200 to 12,000 milligrams of vitamin C a day, which is roughly the same as eating between 45 and 170 oranges.

I do not suggest that you take megadoses of vitamin C as Dr. Pauling did. A recent study has shown a link between high doses of vitamin C pills and hardening of the arteries. However, I do suggest that you begin taking a supplement to be sure that your body is getting plenty of vitamin C. Vitamin C is commonly understood to be a vitamin that will easily flush from your body if you take too much. Therefore be sure you get at least the recommended daily allowance or more. And try to get as much of your vitamin C from your food sources as possible instead of from a pill. Two to 3 grams daily is considered adequate to combat the ravages of aging.[10]

INCREASE YOUR STAYING
POWER WITH VITAMIN E

Supplementing your diet with vitamin E has been proven to slow the aging process in your body.[11] But vitamin E has other benefits as well. It has been shown to boost immunity.[12] In addition, it helps protect your body against heart disease.[13] Vitamin E is also valuable in cancer prevention, and it helps strengthen the body to combat the ravages of rheumatoid arthritis.[14] Individuals with Alzheimer's disease were able to maintain mental function longer when given vitamin E. Vitamin E also reduces the risk of memory loss that can result from the aging process.[15]

Vitamin E slows the aging process in several ways.

+ It helps the body protect itself against the oxidative damage of DNA in cells.[16] If you remember, I discussed earlier how aging tends to cause DNA to break down in cells that are being reproduced. Vitamin E helps to keep this from occurring.

+ Vitamin E also helps to inhibit LDL oxidation.[17] LDL is bad cholesterol in the blood that turns rancid when it meets with oxygen. This process leads to hardening of the arteries. However, supplementing your diet with vitamin E can keep this oxidation from taking place.

+ Vitamin E also helps the body to transport vital glucose throughout the cells and helps to regulate cell growth.[18] We have already discussed how aging takes place at a cellular level. If the body does not have the materials it needs to reproduce cells efficiently, then the next

generation of cells will be less perfect than the
previous one. As this continues to occur in the
cells of the skin, organs, and other parts of the
body, the effects of aging, such as wrinkled
skin, begin to manifest. By helping the body
replenish cells, aging is slowed. Vitamin E can
keep your skin looking younger!

Vitamin E is found in fat-soluble foods such as vegetable oils (primarily soybean, sunflower, and corn oils), nuts,
seeds, whole grains, and wheat germ. It is also in some vegetables. If you are under thirty-five years of age, you can get
all the vitamin E you need in a very healthy diet by supplementing with a multivitamin/mineral daily. However, it is
virtually impossible to get age-retarding doses of vitamin E
in your food.

If you are over thirty-five years of age, take at least 100 to
400 international units (IU) of vitamin E daily. Take vitamin E
with meals, and if possible, take it a couple of times a day rather
than once. This will keep the blood levels consistently high. As a
word of caution, do not take more than 1,000 IU daily.

BEAT THE AGING RAP
WITH BETA-CAROTENE

Taking vitamin C and E will help save you from premature
aging. But you won't get the maximum antiaging effect without
also getting lots of beta-carotene.

Beta-carotene is the orange pigment found in carrots and
other vegetables. This antioxidant fills in where other vitamins
and antioxidants leave off. Beta-carotene is a powerful force
against cancer, heart disease, cataracts, and failing immunity—
in other words, the general deterioration caused by aging.[19]
When individuals suffering from senile dementia were tested,

researchers discovered that they often had a very low intake of beta-carotene as compared to those who continued to have sharp mental abilities throughout old age.[20]

Beta-carotene is found in carrots, sweet potatoes, pumpkin, apricots, broccoli, and spinach. If you are under thirty-five years of age, eating a diet plentiful in these vegetables and fruits will provide all the beta-carotene your body needs. If you are older than thirty-five, you may choose to begin supplementing your diet with a daily supplement of 15,000 to 25,000 IU of beta-carotene to be sure you are getting all of this vital substance your body requires to slow the aging process.

THE THREEFOLD PUNCH

Taking vitamin C, vitamin E, and beta-carotene supplements can produce a threefold supplement cocktail that will dramatically set back the effects of aging.

As mentioned earlier, free radicals are molecular shrapnel caused by the damaging effects of oxygen on the cells. Many researchers strongly believe that free radicals alone contribute to much of what we call aging at a cellular level. Others feel that free radicals, together with the many other factors we have already discussed, all combine to cause aging.

Whatever you believe about aging and free radicals, there is little doubt that free radicals have a dramatic impact on the aging process. You can receive help in staving off aging from any one of the three supplements I have mentioned: vitamin C, vitamin E, and beta-carotene. Each one individually packs plenty of antioxidant power for fighting off bodily deterioration due to free radicals. But the effect of all three taken together is drastically increased.[21]

Here is what Harvard researchers found in studies of thousands of female nurses. In women getting lots of vitamin E, mostly from supplements (more than 200 IU daily), the odds of major cardiovascular disease dropped 34 percent. Those who took high amounts of beta-carotene reduced their risk of heart disease by 22 percent. Female nurses taking high dosages of vitamin C reduced the odds 20 percent. But in women getting the highest amounts of all three antioxidants, the risk of heart disease dropped nearly 50 percent.[22]

The same holds true for cancer and strokes as well. This cumulative antioxidant effect from all three is far better than any single antioxidant at slowing the steady clogging and deterioration of the arteries, thus preventing heart attacks and strokes.[23]

B VITAMINS AND FOLIC ACID

It makes little sense not to take a daily B vitamin supplement that contains B_{12}, B_6, and folic acid. Folic acid also occurs abundantly in fresh, leafy green vegetables. A deficiency of B vitamins in your blood levels—deficiencies that are often undetectable when tested—can cause your body to begin to display symptoms of senility or, worse, Alzheimer's disease. One major study showed that 28 percent of patients with neurological disturbances with no signs of anemia attributable to B_{12} deficiency still suffered dementia, loss of balance, and other psychiatric disorders due to a lack of vitamin B_{12}.[24]

According to research by Tufts University, if you don't get enough B_6, you may become more vulnerable to the classic signs of aging: a failing immune system, declining mental sharpness, a weak heart, and a compromised immune system.[25]

Breakthrough research shows that folic acid helps to direct the growth of new cells in the body as a traffic cop might direct traffic. A shortage or lack of folic acid may result in abnormal cells. It is widely known that a lack of folic acid in the early stages of pregnancy increases the chances of birth defects.

Since aging is very much involved in the faulty reproduction of cells, getting enough folic acid is a must.

Recent studies showed that taking more than the recommended dietary allowance of folic acid and vitamin B_6 may be an important way of preventing coronary heart disease.[26] Experimental results link higher intake of folic acid and vitamin B_{12} with lower homocysteine levels.[27] Epidemiological observations also suggest a strong association between elevated homocysteine levels and cardiovascular disease.[28]

People who puff twenty to thirty cigarettes a day are likely to cough up mucus or phlegm containing precancerous cells. When these precancerous cells become malignant, full-blown lung cancer results. Eliminating these precancerous cells could reduce the incidence of cancer. This is what happened when researchers at the University of Alabama gave smokers very high doses of folic acid and vitamin B_{12}. Amazingly, large numbers of premalignant cells just disappeared within four months, even though the people kept smoking.[29] This provided powerful proof that, in addition to other amazing benefits, B vitamins hold incredible cancer-fighting properties too!

If you are over sixty years of age, it is safest to take doses of no more than the following:

+ 50 milligrams of B_6 daily

+ 400–1,000 micrograms of folic acid daily

+ 500–1,000 micrograms of B_{12} daily

To make it easy, just take a B vitamin supplement daily, regardless of your age.

THE POWER OF VITAMINS

We eat so that our bodies can have the vitamins and energy we need. Too many of us have remained ignorant about the vital role that vitamins play in the health and longevity of our bodies, and we have been robbed of much as a result. The Lord proclaimed through the ancient prophet Hosea, "My people are destroyed for lack of knowledge" (Hosea 4:6, KJV).

Don't let a lack of knowledge about vital vitamins shorten your life span. By giving your body all that it needs to function at its best, you will be like the Energizer bunny. When your peers are beginning to slow down, you will keep going and going and going!

Chapter 7

MINING MINERALS FOR LONGEVITY

*And the LORD God formed
man of the dust of the ground.*

—GENESIS 2:7

I F VITAMINS ARE the gasoline for the antiaging engine, then minerals are the oil. The Bible says that our bodies were originally created from the dust of the ground, which is why they contain the same minerals as soil. "Then the LORD God formed man from the dust of the ground and breathed into his nostrils the breath of life, and man became a living being" (Gen. 2:7, MEV).

Because we were created from dust, all the materials that form us are found in the earth. Of the elements most important for our organs to function and survive, minerals top the list, and we obtain them, directly or indirectly, from soil. No plant or animal survives without them. The planets and stars are made of them, and we humans desperately need them in our earthly bodies.

Minerals allow the body to keep a balance between acidity and alkalinity. Our bodies require minerals because they are continuously rebuilding themselves. This function is carried out in each one of the cells, and minerals and vitamins act as catalyzing agents in the process. When these catalysts are lacking, the biochemical reactions are carried out in an incomplete way, forming toxic products that slow down the regeneration process.

When denied essential minerals, our bodies experience degeneration, which is part of the aging process. The foods that the average North American eats do not maintain the body's mineral supply at an adequate level. The human body has neither the power to extract minerals directly from the environment nor the ability to manufacture them from other substances. Our only source of mineral provision is food. Some of the foods that provide the best supply of minerals are broccoli, spinach, watercress, coriander, lettuce, parsley, sweet peppers, tomatoes, chili peppers, prickly pears, and mushrooms.

United States government surveys confirm that the average American diet provides only 40 percent of the recommended daily amount of magnesium. A two-year Food and Drug Administration study analyzing 234 foods found that the average American diet has less than 80 percent of the recommended daily allowance (RDA) of one or more of the following minerals: calcium, magnesium, iron, zinc, copper, and manganese. What makes this worse is the fact that RDAs are sadly insufficient for maintaining health.

A large study conducted by the United States Department of Agriculture (USDA) found that only 25 percent of 37,785 individuals had magnesium intakes at or greater than the RDA, which is notoriously low. A 1995 review of fifteen studies found that a typical diet contains only a fraction of the RDA.[1]

Let's look at some minerals essential in the fight to reverse the aging process.

THE POWER OF CHROMIUM

Rats given chromium picolinate continued to live and thrive for a full year beyond their normal life expectancy—which was a full one-third longer.[2] In humans that would increase the average life span from 75 years to 102 years!

Gary Evans, PhD, a professor of chemistry at Minnesota State University in Bemidji, Minnesota, and a prominent chromium researcher, said, "I wasn't surprised. I expected them to live longer because they had many of the characteristics of lab animals on restricted-calorie diets, and those animals always live longer."[3] The mechanism by which chromium picolinate prolongs life is possibly by regulating the blood levels of glucose and lipids.

If you are age twenty or older, chances are that you lack chromium and will therefore age much faster than you need to.[4] Most of us do not get enough chromium in our diets. In addition, the levels of chromium in our bodies decrease with age.

When you take a chromium supplement every day, your body will be helped in a number of ways:

+ Body fat decreases when chromium is added to the diet.

+ Lean muscle tissue is improved, and "bad cholesterol" (LDL) is reduced.[5]

The most important reason to take chromium is to save yourself from accelerated aging brought on by too much of the hormone insulin in your blood. Too much insulin can bring about diabetes and can destroy your arteries. One-fourth of Americans past middle age have a serious insulin disorder.[6]

Dr. Evans said, "I call chromium the 'geriatric nutrient,' because everybody starts to really need it past age thirty-five."[7]

So, how much chromium should you take? Here is my recommendation: after age thirty-five, take at least 200 to 500 micrograms of chromium per day.

MIGHTY SELENIUM

In addition to needing more chromium, most individuals have far too little selenium in their diets. This remarkable mineral has a dramatic effect on all the known aging mechanisms. Populations whose diets contain a lot of selenium live longer. And conversely, populations whose diets are deficient in selenium have a reduced life span.[8] The possible reason for the elevated mortality in selenium-deficient areas may be accelerated aging due to excessive cellular damage caused by oxygen-free radicals.

This wonderful mineral strengthens the body against heart disease and other chronic illnesses such as cancer.[9] Selenium can also help keep viruses, even vicious ones like HIV, which produces AIDS, from breaking out of cells and spreading destruction throughout the body. When your cells get low on selenium, as they tend to do when you age, your immune system functioning is negatively impacted.[10]

As you grow older, the level of selenium in your body is reduced. After age sixty, selenium levels fall 7 percent, and after age seventy-five, selenium levels plummet 24 percent. People with less selenium in their blood have more heart disease, cancer, and arthritis.[11]

If you are over age forty, take 200 to 400 micrograms of selenium daily for the maximum antiaging effect. A single Brazil nut contains the same amount of selenium as a selenium pill, but the nut must be one from a shell. The average Brazil nut contains about 100 micrograms of selenium, and it also has essential fatty acids!

THE POTENCY OF ZINC

Zinc is one of the most important trace elements in your body for many vital biological functions, including DNA and protein synthesis, cell division, and gene expression. Zinc is an integral component for more than two hundred enzymes, many proteins, hormones, neuropeptides, hormone receptors, and other biological structures. Due to these important physiological roles zinc is considered a major element in assuring the correct functioning of your body, from your very first embryonic stages to the last days of your life.[12]

If there was ever a mineral connected to a biological clock, zinc would be it. Zinc is closely related to the working of a little gland behind the top of the breastbone called the thymus. When you were born, your thymus was bigger than your heart. But by the time you were forty, it was almost impossible to find on an X-ray.[13]

The thymus, the primary organ of the immune system, is therefore called the pacemaker of aging.[14] With the shrinkage of the thymus comes increasingly reduced levels of zinc. As the body is more and more depleted of zinc, the ability of the immune system to fend off the ravages of aging is greatly diminished.

However, it is possible to reverse this process. Experiments in rodents in which dietary zinc was supplemented demonstrated that many age-related immune system changes could be reversed. Amazingly, taking zinc supplements even caused the thymus to regrow.[15]

French researchers discovered that even in the very elderly, immune systems can be salvaged by supplementing zinc. These scientists gave a group of institutionalized people, aged 73 to 106 years, 20 milligrams of zinc daily, and the activity of their thymus glands shot up as much as 50 percent within a couple of months. Almost all of the subjects were deficient in zinc to begin with.

Interestingly, increasing levels of zinc caused blood levels of albumin, a protein notoriously low in most elderly persons, to rise as well. Albumin is a biomarker of longevity—those with high levels live longer! Thus, zinc may indirectly extend life.[16]

If you are over thirty-five years of age, take a daily dose of 15 to 30 milligrams of zinc. However, if you are over seventy-five, you may need a dose of 50 milligrams or more to substantially retrieve thymus activity. Such high doses should not be taken without careful medical supervision.[17]

A MULTIMINERAL SOLUTION

Maureen Kennedy Salaman, author of *Foods That Heal* and *All Your Health Questions Answered Naturally*, is an authority on the subject of minerals. She recommends taking a mineral solution supplemental formula. Salaman says, "Minerals in solution are easily assimilated into the body, and are not compromised by allergies, digestive problems or a lack of stomach acid."[18] I agree with her; taking minerals in solution will help you to absorb them better.

THE NATURAL POWER OF NUTRIENTS

Now that we have taken a look at some minerals that can powerfully impact how you age and how long you live, let's look at some other nutrients that have proven powerfully effective in combating the aging process.

Coenzyme Q_{10}

One of the main complaints of aging is diminished energy at a cellular level. Coenzyme Q_{10} can help.

Just as your car's engine needs a spark to get going, the cells of your body need a similar kind of spark. Coenzyme Q_{10} provides the spark that starts the mitochondria engines. Free radicals rob energy production by attacking mitochondria. This is the part of cells where oxygen is burned to give the cells enough energy to carry on the business of life. Without this spark, cell life, as well as all human life, would cease to exist.[19]

Coenzyme Q_{10} is a naturally occurring fat-soluble quinone with vitamin-like properties, which is an essential component of the energy production process that takes place in the mitochondria of the cells. As an antioxidant, coenzyme Q_{10} plays an important role in protecting heart mitochondria from the damage of free radicals during aging.[20] It also inhibits LDL oxidation ("bad cholesterol") and aids in preventing atherosclerosis.[21]

As you get older, your body's reserves of coenzyme Q_{10} decline. The level of coenzyme Q_{10} also decreases significantly in smokers and those with high cholesterol levels and heart disease. Evidence exists linking cancer with low levels of coenzyme Q_{10}, together with immune system dysfunction.[22]

We have already seen that the aging process is associated with an increase in cellular oxidation. This may be due in part to a decline in the levels of coenzyme Q_{10}. This nutrient can also be applied topically to reduce the impact of aging on the skin.[23]

If you are over forty, here is my advice: Take 50 milligrams daily of a commercially available form of coenzyme Q_{10} with your heaviest meal. Or take 30 milligrams a day of a new fully soluble form of coenzyme Q_{10} (Q-Gel) that possesses a high bioavailability (2.73-fold higher than the commercial forms).[24]

Brain-enhancing and heart-protecting fish oils

Fish oils contain two omega-3 fatty acids called EPA and DHA. However, plants provide a rich source of another omega-3 fatty acid called alpha-linolenic acid (ALA).

Studies of Eskimos and the Japanese—who both consume large quantities of fish and other marine life rich in fish oils—have shown that both groups have a far lower risk of suffering from cardiovascular disease, which is the major cause of early death.[25] Taking supplemental DHA in the diet improves learning ability, whereas deficiencies of DHA are associated with deficits in learning.[26] Decreases in DHA in the brain are related with cognitive decline during aging and with onset of sporadic Alzheimer's disease.[27]

You can increase your intake of omega-3 fatty acids in the following ways:

+ Eat fatty fish. Fish with the most antiaging omega-3 oils (EPA and DHA) are mackerel, anchovies, herring, salmon, sardines, halibut, and bass. Fish with moderate amounts are turbot, bluefish, tuna, striped bass, smelt, oysters, swordfish, bass, rainbow trout, and pompano.[28]

+ Eat vegetable oils. Canola and soybean oils are rich sources of ALA.[29]

+ Eat plant foods with relatively high content in omega-3 (ALA), such as nuts, seeds, and soybeans.[30]

+ Take flaxseed oil as a supplement. This oil is particularly rich in omega-3 fatty acids, mainly ALA with an average content of 58 percent.[31]

Dietary omega-3 fatty acids reduce coronary heart disease risk by lowering total blood cholesterol without decreasing HDL ("good" cholesterol) levels,[32] preventing fatal cardiac arrhythmia,[33] inhibiting atherosclerosis,[34] and inhibiting clotting.[35]

In one study 20,551 male physicians were followed up for eleven years to explore the link between fish consumption and the risk of sudden cardiac death. Researchers found that by eating more than one meal with fatty fish a week, the risk of sudden heart attack death decreased 52 percent when compared to eating less than one fish meal per month. Overall mortality risk was also reduced in those who ate fish frequently.[36] The most powerful cardiovascular disease action of omega-3 fatty acids from both fish and plants is that it actually helps to prevent ventricular fibrillation and sudden death.

If you have never had heart disease, then consume 2–3 grams of fish oil (equivalent to 0.6–0.9 grams of EPA+DHA) per day for prevention. Higher doses should be used for those who have suffered heart attacks (after myocardial infarction).[37]

ANTIAGING HERBS

The Bible extols the virtues of herbs. It says, "He [God] causeth the grass to grow for the cattle, and herb for the service of man: that he may bring forth food out of the earth" (Ps. 104:14, KJV).

Here are several herbs to add to your shopping list of antiaging supplements.

Garlic

First on the list is garlic. This herb has been known for its medicinal properties for centuries, but it is best known for its spicy zest. Aged garlic extract has the ability to prolong life span, improve learning and spatial memory, and prevent the physical changes in the brain connected with aging in mice.[38]

Japanese researcher Dr. Hiroshi Saito, professor of pharmaceutical sciences at the University of Tokyo, screened dozens of natural and synthetic products searching for a new treatment for senility. He has proven that garlic extract reduces the old-age-related destruction of rat brain cells, and even more startling, it stimulates the branching of new brain neurons. Saito says that garlic helps to ensure brain cell survival into old age and even helps old brains to regenerate or actually grow younger.[39]

Garlic has many other life-extending properties. It can be used to prevent arteriosclerosis,[40] to protect against cardiovascular disease,[41] to prevent cancer,[42] to inhibit and/or scavenge oxygen free radicals[43] and to combat microbes.[44]

Much of garlic's activity derives from alliin and allicin (or its immediate by-products such as S-allyl-cysteine and S-allyl-mercaptocysteine found in aged garlic extracts). In addition, garlic contains the minerals selenium and tellurium.[45]

The aged garlic used in Dr. Saito's experiments is called "Kyolic." From one-half to two or three fresh cloves a day should give your cells a youth-saving injection. Two to three fresh garlic cloves equal:

- 1 teaspoon of garlic powder

- Four 1-gram tablets (1,000 milligrams) of powdered garlic such as Kwai

- Four gel caps of Kyolic garlic

- 1 teaspoon of liquid Kyolic garlic

In supplements, 600 to 1,200 milligrams of active garlic powder per day have produced documented heart-protective effects.

Ginkgo biloba

Ginkgo biloba has been used for several thousand years in Chinese traditional medicine for treating asthma and bronchitis. The ginkgo biloba tree is one of the oldest living things on earth; it can live almost four thousand years.

This amazing tree also appears to produce substances that can help us to live longer. Lab rats who were given ginkgo biloba extended their lives almost 20 percent.[46] In Europe ginkgo biloba is prescribed as a drug for the treatment of senility and dementia (Alzheimer's disease) and for a variety of symptoms associated with aging.[47]

Ginkgo biloba extract increases mental efficiency and improves memory loss in elderly persons.[48] In addition, research has proven that ginkgo biloba is very effective in the treatment of both erectile dysfunction and sexual dysfunction linked to the use of antidepressants.[49]

Ginkgo biloba leaves and fruit contain flavonoids and a collection of unusual substances called *terpenoids* (ginkgolides) that are unique in the vegetable kingdom. These possess amazing antioxidant power by acting as free-radical scavengers and by inhibiting the formation of free radicals.[50]

Based on current research, here is a list of the powerful things this superherb can do:

+ Improve blood flow, especially in deeper-seated medium and small arteries in vital organs such as the brain and heart

+ Improve failing memory and information processing

+ Slow the progression of Alzheimer's disease

+ Reduce leg pain from lack of blood flow

+ Inhibit bacterial activity of gum disease

+ Relieve vertigo or dizziness

+ Reduce ringing in the ears (tinnitus)

+ Inhibit deteriorating vision due to oxygen deprivation of the retina

+ Improve hearing loss related to blood flow

+ Raise HDL (good cholesterol)

+ Inhibit abnormal blood clotting

+ Lower blood pressure

+ Relieve male impotence by promoting blood flow

+ Relieve Raynaud's disease, a circulatory disease
  resulting in cold hands and feet

Nearly all scientific studies have used a standardized form of ginkgo called EGb 761, which is made in Germany. It is sold in tablet form in the United States under the name "Ginkgold." The normal dosage is one 60-milligram tablet twice a day. Drinking tea made from ginkgo leaves will not provide the same benefits as taking the tablet twice a day.

Panax ginseng

Another popular Asian herb has netted surprising results in the battle against aging. Panax ginseng, whose active components include complex glycosides known as ginsenoides, is well tested, for it has been used in China for the past two thousand years.

Research has shown that ginseng extract scavenges the blood of free radicals that produce hardening of the arteries and possibly cancer. This antioxidant effect is also believed to be responsible for ginseng's antiaging effect.[51]

Here are some other dramatic effects:

+ Reduces fatigue[52]

+ Fights tumors[53]

+ Helps with concentration, memory, and mental alertness[54]

+ Helps protect cardiovascular system

+ Helps the body to resist the stress of environmental pollution

+ Improves erectile dysfunction[55]

Panax ginseng, which is also known as Chinese or Korean ginseng, is the most famous ginseng. Check the label of your ginseng product before purchasing it for its ginsenoside content. Your dosage of ginseng is related to how much ginsenoside your selection contains. For example, if you are taking a high-quality root powder or extract containing 5 to 7 percent ginsenosides, the dosage would be 100 milligrams twice daily.

Grape seed extract

Exciting advances in research have revealed that grape seed extract (proanthocyanidin) can help your skin look younger much longer, as well as help your body fight off many assaults of aging.

Grapes are one of the most widely consumed fruits in the world, and they are rich in proanthocyanidins, which are natural flavonoids with extraordinary properties. More than 60 percent of these flavonoids are found in the grape seeds.

Grape seed extract contains many cancer-fighting properties. It also helps your body to fight inflammation, arthritis, allergies, and heart disease. Research has shown that skin tends to age more slowly when you take grape seed extract.[56] In addition, taking grape seed proanthocyanidins also significantly improves vision and strengthens other organs, such as the liver and brain.[57]

The dosage for grape seed extract is 100 to 150 milligrams daily.

Barleygreen

Barleygreen is one of the most powerful whole-food supplements I know of. It is a multipurpose product that I have been taking myself for years. It is a powdered substance developed by Dr. Yoshihide Hagiwara, a Japanese pharmacologist and physician. As a grain, barley has outstanding nutritional value. It contains chlorophyll, enzymes, minerals, amino acids, and vitamins, and it is packed with phytochemicals that help the body detoxify itself from built-up poisons and heavy metals.

The genius of Dr. Hagiwara's product is what he does to the soil before the barley is planted. He believes that tired and depleted soil, which he calls dead soil, produces dead plants. His agriculture specialists prepare barleygreen soil with nutrients, not with chemical fertilizers. Since the Japanese have the longest life span of any other industrialized country, I value their nutritional knowledge and research.

CONCLUSION:
WISDOM FOR LONGEVITY

Wisdom and good sense are required to care for our bodies, wisdom that will yield powerful benefits as we begin to age.

Wisdom is knowledge put into practice. Knowledge alone is worthless. Solomon said that the beginning of wisdom is the fear of the Lord (Prov. 9:10). You may ask, "What does that have to do with what minerals and nutrients I take?" The fear of the Lord has nothing to do with being afraid of Him; it has everything to do with respecting Him as the Creator. Creation requires law to maintain order. We are, like it or not, still subject to the rules of the game. In other words, the laws of nature cannot be broken without exacting a toll. And often that toll is premature aging and early death.

In God's divine wisdom He created our bodies to function by being properly fueled with a vast array of essential minerals and nutrients. We honor the wisdom of God's laws by caring for our bodies with awesome respect for His creative genius. The benefits of obeying these wise laws are renewed vigor, rejuvenated health, and increased longevity.

Chapter 8

DISCOVERING ENZYMES
AND HORMONES

*You're not old until you
have lost all of your marvels.*

—ANONYMOUS

A CONCEPT OF GOD that church fathers came up with many years ago says that God is a God of infinity, both of the macrocosmically infinite and the microcosmically infinite. What that means is that we are surrounded by eternity, both in terms of what is larger than we are and what is smaller than we are. A look into space reveals a macrocosmic infinity. It seems that as far as we can go or can even imagine, the universe stretches out beyond us.

But another universe exists beyond us as well. It is the universe that stretches out infinitely beyond our vision because of its smallness: the microcosmic infinity.

God has not simply written His creative signature in trees, mountains, brooks, oceans, and rivers. God has spoken to us about Himself as an eternal being by placing us in a world surrounded by infinity.

Our ancestors sailed oceans and discovered continents in fulfillment of God's command to be fruitful and to fill the earth and subdue it. (See Genesis 1:28.) To subdue the earth, adventurers risked their lives on flimsy vessels to locate and chart the world beyond them. But today adventurers strain through shadowy instruments, peering into the microcosmic infinity to do the very same thing.

The mysteries of lands and continents, oceans and mountains gave up their secrets to our ancestors. But it is the microcosmic world that holds the secrets of aging—secrets that scientists and adventurers long to understand and subdue.

We have taken a look at the mysteries of this cellular universe by discussing vitamins, minerals, DNA, and the impact of such things on aging. Let's strain our eyes a little more and look a little deeper still into this mysterious microcosmic universe with these modern-day adventurers to get a glimpse of another key to aging: the work of enzymes and hormones. Of all the agents for prolonging life, hormones are the most complex and difficult to apply without controversy and risk. We shall limit our discussion of enzymes only to telomerase, which holds promises for prolonging life.

LENGTHENING TIME'S TAIL
WITH TELOMERASE

Telomerase is an enzyme that holds powerful promise in cracking the code of aging.

As we mentioned earlier, each of our chromosomes has a long tail called the telomere. Beginning in the 1960s scientists theorized that these telomeres act as a cellular clock. Each time the cell divides, the telomere acts as a burning fuse, shortening each time until the telomere runs out and the cell starts to die.[1]

Scientists believe they have discovered an enzyme called telomerase that rebuilds the continuously changing length of the body's telomeres. This means that if the burning fuse causes aging, then scientists can actually begin to reverse the aging process at its very source. What is particularly exciting is that when skin, retinal, and vascular cells in the laboratory were triggered to produce telomerase, the internal clocks of these cells were rewound and the cells lived much longer than normal.

These scientists believe that they are the first to extend the life of human cells. Others have done so, only they have harmed cells in the process, such as turning the cells cancerous. When cells were engineered to produce telomerase, which older cells do not do, they continued to divide rapidly.[2] According to early reports, the telomerase-engineered cells lived almost twice as long as normal.[3] This means that in the future it might be possible to extend our lives by lengthening the life spans of our individual cells one by one.

Telomerase and cancer

Unlike normal human cells, cancer cells do not die. They replicate so rapidly that they form tumors. The telomerase theory got another shot in the arm by the discovery that cancer cells contain telomerase. Researchers concluded that it was the telomerase in the cancer cells that caused them to keep replicating.

Researchers surmised that if they understood what caused cancer cells to live on endlessly, they could then make some cellular adjustments that might force the cancer cells to die. This kind of research is going on right now.

Other promises

The discovery of telomerase promises even more tremendous breakthroughs. Cells that die cause many diseases, from muscular dystrophy to arteriosclerosis. Telomerase might be able to keep those cells from dying, either through gene therapy inside the body or by altering cells in a lab and injecting them back into a patient.[4]

A flood of opposition and mixed reviews

Just when researchers thought they had cracked a significant code to aging and disease, a flood of opposition created enough skepticism to cool the fires of enthusiasm—at least temporarily.

Opponents of the research created mice that were deficient in telomerase and bred them, creating five generations of the gene-deficient creatures. When the mice were injected with cancer cells, they got cancer. The researchers theorized that either the cancer cells can override the telomerase-deficient chromosomes and continue dividing, or the cancer has more than one way to repair telomere damage.[5]

But other scientists disagree with these conclusions, arguing that mice and people develop cancer in such different ways that such a conclusion is not possible to make. In addition, mouse telomeres are much longer than human ones, which could have affected the test results.

So the jury is still out on telomerase. The promise of the enzyme telomerase is powerful, but research is still in the infant stage. It is possible, though, that this enzyme may be a significant key to cracking the code of aging.

THE PROMISE OF
HUMAN GROWTH HORMONE

Hormones are trace substances produced by various endocrine glands. They serve as chemical messengers carried by the blood to various target organs, where they regulate a variety of physical and metabolic activities.

All infants are born with a significant amount of growth hormone in their pituitary glands. The pituitary gland, located at the base of the brain, is called a master gland in the body because it sends many different hormones throughout the body to function in numerous ways. One of the primary hormones it produces is the growth hormone, which regulates growth.

Growth hormone decreases with age, which impacts aging in many ways. Lower levels of this hormone are linked to decreased lean body and bone mass, increased body fat, and the loss of tissue functions, such as elasticity of the skin. The lower levels of this hormone in aging also make it more difficult for the body to use proteins.[6]

Hormones have many dramatic effects on the body, and the impact of growth hormone is absolutely no different. Growth hormone slows down and reverses many of the aging processes that occur in older individuals. It also reverses many of the problems that are caused by aging, such as wrinkled skin, increased body fat, decreased muscle mass, increased cholesterol, decreased stamina and energy, and decreased mental function.[7]

Not long ago researchers began experimenting with this marvelous hormone in mice. Their tests yielded some interesting and hopeful results. In an experiment at North Dakota State University elderly mice (nineteen months old) were injected with either growth hormone or saline twice a week. After thirteen weeks 39 percent of the saline mice were still alive, which is normal according to the mice's life expectancy. However, 93 percent of the mice that received growth hormone were still alive. In other words, the life expectancy of the growth-hormone mice was off the charts!

When the injections were stopped for six weeks, all of the remaining saline mice died of old age. But only one of the twenty remaining growth-hormone mice died. So the researchers started giving these nineteen remaining mice growth hormone again for another six weeks. Do you know what happened? At the end of the six-week period eighteen of the mice, now living far beyond their normal life expectancy, remained alive.[8]

When elderly humans were given growth hormone, they were affected in some very interesting ways. Their muscle mass increased, bones became more dense, and their skin became thicker, to name a few of the startling results.[9]

Dr. Lawrence Dorman, of Kansas City, Missouri, a member of the American Academy of Antiaging, expressed great excitement over the hormone treatment results. "I attended the Antiaging Conference with over one thousand other physicians from around the world. Most doctors who attended agreed that Human Growth Hormone was one of the most exciting advancements in reversing the disease process since DHEA," said Dr. Dorman.[10]

Growth hormone can be stimulated in young adults by weight training and resistance exercises. Aerobic exercise can also have a profound effect in stimulating growth hormone production in individuals over forty years of age.[11]

The sellers of synthetic, orally administered growth hormone treatments boast everything from increased muscle mass to hair regrowth. As long as the correct amounts are taken, no negative side effects should be experienced—at least that is what the manufacturers say.[12] Injections and orally administered hormone treatments are available by prescription.

However, though research has netted some positive results, the jury is still out on taking growth hormone supplements. Although some researchers are sold on the positive effects of synthetic growth hormones, other researchers refute the tests. Therefore it is probably best to wait until more test results validate the promise of synthetic growth hormone. If you are too eager to wait, at least be very careful to take the right dosage. Taking too much can produce extremely negative side effects, such as men growing large breasts and both men and women getting arthritis and retaining fluid, and carpal tunnel syndrome.[13]

Another hormone is safer to use, easier to get, less expensive, and better tested. It is melatonin.

THE MIRACLE OF MELATONIN

Melatonin is a hormone produced by the pineal gland and is thought to work as a centralized clock to help regulate sleep and aging. During infancy and childhood a high degree of melatonin reaches every cell. This high level lets the cells know that the organism is young. Proteins that are needed for growth and repair are then manufactured. As an individual ages, the amount of melatonin is gradually lessened. Therefore, as we advance in years, less and less melatonin reaches the DNA in our cells.[14]

Over the years the declining levels of melatonin send the cells information about your body's age. That is why some researchers believe that supplementing melatonin could trick your body's DNA into thinking that you are younger than you really are. Melatonin inhibits free-radical damage to DNA caused by ionizing radiation, chemical carcinogens, and environmental toxic agents.[15] Melatonin can help repair DNA and can prevent the damage to DNA caused by chemicals. As a result of taking melatonin, your body could experience fewer age-related changes, leaving you with younger skin, younger organs, more energy, and best of all, a longer life span.

Melatonin might also work to prolong life by supporting the immune system, acting as a free-radical scavenger, stimulating some important antioxidative enzymes (such as superoxide dismutase), and stabilizing cell membranes, thereby making them more resistant to oxidative attack.[16]

Interestingly, melatonin may even be linked to the fantastic life extension results discovered through food restriction. Food restriction in rodents causes their levels of melatonin to rise. We have already discussed the life-extending powers that result from food restriction experiments. Researchers say that it is too early to tell if the increase in melatonin due to food restriction is what actually causes this increased longevity. When the test results are in, they promise to be powerfully revealing.[17]

Mice and melatonin

In other tests researchers found that when middle-aged male mice were given melatonin in their drinking water nightly, they tended to live an average of 20 percent longer. Researchers reported, "To our surprise, chronic, nightly administration of melatonin resulted in a progressive, striking improvement of the general state of the mice and, most important, in a remarkable prolongation of their lives."[18] Interestingly, five months after the mice began receiving melatonin, the mice appeared astonishingly healthier, more active, and more vigorous than those not getting melatonin.[19]

However, when melatonin was fed to female, premenopausal mice, the results were exactly the opposite. Melatonin shortened their life span by 6 percent.[20] In addition, many of these mice experienced ovarian cancer. The age of these mice would correspond to thirty-five years old in a human. But different mouse strains reacted much differently, even to these tests, and the amount they received factored for body weight was much higher than what a human would receive.

When female mice who had already reached menopause were given melatonin, they did not display ovarian cancer and did live 20 percent longer than regular mice.[21]

Melatonin and sleep

Melatonin can profoundly impact an individual's ability to sleep well. As darkness falls, the pineal gland releases a surge of melatonin that begins preparing the body for sleep. When morning light hits the retina of the eye, the pineal gland is signaled to halt the production of melatonin.[22]

Studies show that low doses of melatonin can hasten sleep and ease jet lag without the dangerous side effects of prescription sleeping pills.[23] The lower levels of melatonin in the elderly is no doubt the reason that many older folks suffer from bouts of sleeplessness and many others report sleeping irregularly or too lightly to wake up completely refreshed.

Researchers have found low levels of melatonin in individuals who suffer with insomnia. Treating insomniacs with low doses of melatonin for seven days can improve sleep patterns in elderly patients.[24] Young adults report deeper sleep after such melatonin treatments.[25]

More about melatonin

Melatonin has also proven itself as a powerful antioxidant, which helps rid the body of potential cancer-causing materials.[26] In addition, it helps the body to fight heart disease by decreasing bad cholesterol (or decreasing the atherogenic uptake of LDL) and helping to normalize blood pressure.[27] In experimental models used to study changes to the brain caused by Alzheimer's and Parkinson's disease, melatonin was also found to be effective in protecting against nervous system damage caused by free radicals.[28]

Melatonin must be taken before going to bed. If you are between forty and fifty years old, take 0.5 to 1.0 milligram. If you are fifty to sixty years old, take 1 to 2 milligrams, and if you are between sixty and seventy years old, take 2 to 3 milligrams before going to bed. Those over seventy years old should take 3 milligrams.

There is little doubt that hormones like melatonin produce a powerful effect. But opponents argue that the benefits of melatonin have been exaggerated. However, even those who are strongly opposed agree that the benefits to the sleepless are beyond dispute. As the research data pile up on this powerful hormone, keep your eye on it. Its promises are too important to dismiss too easily or too soon.

HORMONE REPLACEMENT THERAPIES

We are all familiar with testosterone and estrogen therapies, which are currently available as hormone replacement therapies. Some researchers are beginning to look at these therapies for aging keys.

Testosterone replacement treatments

According to Dr. Gabe Mirkin, author of *The Sports Medicine Book* and *Fat Free, Flavor Full: Dr. Gabe Mirkin's Guide to Losing Weight and Living Longer,* some men can lose some strength, assertiveness, and much of their sexuality as they age. Replacing the declining male sex hormone testosterone can help. From age fifty to seventy, the average man's testosterone level drops by more than 40 percent. Present data from scientific studies suggest there is real potential for testosterone administration to improve bone mass and lean body mass and strength, and to reduce fat mass in old men.[29] Effects on mood, libido, and cognition are less clear but may be meaningful in certain men.[30]

The long-term risks of testosterone therapy on older men really are not known, especially in the areas of cardiovascular disease and benign and malignant prostate disease.[31] One major caution exists, however. Prostate cancer, so common in older men, can spread throughout the body after supplementing testosterone. Therefore, if you decide to ask your doctor for testosterone replacement therapy, just make sure that he checks you carefully for prostate cancer first.

Estrogen and elderly women

Some elderly women take estrogen-replacement therapy to reduce the risks of heart disease and osteoporosis. But most doctors do not prescribe it much beyond menopause because of a risk of developing breast cancer.

However, some doctors feel this risk doesn't override the benefits of estrogen to elderly women. I disagree.

When the menstrual cycle is normal, the ovaries produce the same amount of hormones (at different times) to maintain equilibrium. In normal menopause there is a balance reduction in the production of estrogens and progesterone. However, an estrogenic dominance exists, which not only affects menopausal women but is also the reason why so many suffer premenstrual syndrome and most feminine ailments at all ages.[32]

Conventional practice prescribes synthetic hormone replacement, progesterone in conjunction with estrogens, but such therapies produce serious side effects, including fluid retention, weight gain, depression, allergies, vaginal discharge, nausea, insomnia, and headaches. The answer to this imbalance is natural progesterone. Many other symptoms are resolved through the restoration of hormonal balance as well.[33] Natural progesterone may prolong your life.

Hormones are certainly a major key to aging and to many other functions of the body as well. One hormone seems to act as a bandleader, directing and harmonizing all of the others. It is DHEA.

THE DHEA DEBATE

DHEA (dehydroepiandrosterone), a hormone found in the adrenal glands, goes before all other hormones in the body by supplying what the body needs to maintain a good hormonal balance. As we age, our bodies lose much of their DHEA. These low levels of DHEA are linked to diabetes, obesity, high cholesterol, heart disease, arthritis, and many other symptoms associated with aging.[34]

Many studies have shown that taking supplemental DHEA

can drastically improve mental abilities, such as forgetfulness and memory loss, that often come with aging. DHEA is also believed to help the immune system function better, relieve stress disorders, help the body fight heart disease, and protect against certain forms of cancer.

Sound like a wonder drug? Well, as with growth hormone, the tests look very promising, but the results are not completely conclusive. So once again, it is probably best to take a wait-and-see approach. Nonetheless, research is shining some powerfully bright lights into the area of hormones, what they do for us, and how replacement therapies can help us stave off the negative effects of aging.[35]

In one clinical study at the University of California at San Diego, a dose of 50 milligrams per day of DHEA was administered daily to both men and women. Over a six-month period both men and women said they experienced physical and psychological well-being.[36] Another study, a daily oral dose of 100 milligrams of DHEA for the same period, resulted in decreased fat body mass and increased strength, but selectively in men.[37]

Dr. Arthur Schwartz of Temple University Medical School in Philadelphia said that he carried out a life-span study on mice years ago and found that DHEA was able to thwart hair graying and extend life spans in mice. However, these effects were only observed when the dose of DHEA was high enough to produce unwanted side effects as well.[38] Because of this, Dr. Schwartz began to look for another type of DHEA without the harmful side effects. He claims that he has found it in a fluorinated derivative of DHEA. Not only does it not produce the side effects, but it also helps fight cancer and rodent diabetes and blocks autoimmunity, according to Schwartz.[39]

The testing of DHEA is ongoing and will produce some surprising results. In years to come, you may choose to take

DHEA hormone supplements for everything from weight gain and gray hair to longevity following a heart transplant.

WATCH FOR
DEVELOPMENTS IN HORMONES

The role of hormones is now well determined, but its application is complex. The development of "the pill" by Carl Dejarassi for a Mexican laboratory (Syntex) in the 1960s proved that we could actually play with hormonal interactions and enjoy sex without the risk of pregnancy. But "enjoy" is an exaggeration. It took a few years to uncover the uncomfortable side effects that the majority of women have endured for their sexual freedom. It also took a couple of decades to learn that this hormonal manipulation increased the risk of breast cancer. Estrogen replacement therapy remains under fire because of the risk of developing malignancies, especially of the breast.

While it is true that hormones are involved in the aging process and that hormone manipulation can help us to live longer, the negative impact of this manipulation remains unknown. The problem is the complexity of hormones and the fact that they are extremely potent substances—where minute amounts have major effects. Our bodies deliver hormones sometimes at a steady rate, but more often in a burst according to need. This is extremely difficult, if not impossible, to mimic with medications.

Even though the risk of hormone supplementation can be drastically lessened under the close scrutiny of an endocrinologist and a geriatric specialist, I recommend other means by which you can help your body to enhance its hormonal mechanisms. You can provide your body with all the necessary raw materials needed for hormones to function at their optimum levels through nutrients.

In addition, although some of the greatest breakthroughs in

aging may be years away, you can experience significant anti-aging effects at this very moment. Some of the greatest longevity boosters are just a few sit-ups or push-ups away.

Chapter 9

EXERCISE: GET MOVING TOWARD LONGEVITY!

The older you get, the stronger the wind gets–and it's always in your face.[1]

–JACK NICKLAUS,
US GOLFER

IN CELEBRATION OF his sixtieth birthday, Tommy Barnett—a nationally respected pastor and founder of the Dream Center in Los Angeles—accomplished a feat that most people half his age would not even attempt. Pastor Barnett ran cross-country 426 miles from Phoenix, Arizona, to Los Angeles, California. This 426-mile-run was the fulfillment of a dream that he had had for forty-five years. And he used this cross-country run to raise funds to establish the Dream Center, which touches the lives of inner-city drug addicts, prostitutes, gang members, and the poor.

If you don't believe that exercise has the power to keep you young, just ask Pastor Barnett!

Most of us accelerate the aging process in our bodies with our sedentary lifestyles. Neglecting our bodies through lack of use fuels the ravages of cellular aging just as gasoline feeds a wildfire. But regular, moderate exercise works like a fireman to extinguish the blaze.

You may not be ready to jog across the nation at age sixty, but don't worry. Just being willing to start moving can dramatically change the length and quality of your life, especially in your graying years.

Let's take a closer look at exercise and its impact on your longevity.

According to the Harvard Health Letter, exercise is the best known intervention to ensure that golden years are spent actively and healthily.[2] These experts believe that the nation's fifty-two thousand centenarians reached that milestone largely due to reducing risk factors through healthy lifestyle choices, primarily exercise.[3]

THE TRIUMPH OF VIGOROUS EXERCISE

Vigorous exercise significantly reduces the risk of heart attacks and heart disease. A recent study showed that men who ran the most had lower blood pressure and higher levels of high-density lipoprotein (HDL), which is good cholesterol. Long-term endurance increases longevity by reducing blood pressure, body fat, and bad cholesterol.[4]

A new Harvard study that followed the lives of 17,300 middle-aged men for more than twenty years found that vigorous activities dramatically reduced the risk of dying. The *Journal of the American Medical Association* reported that men who did at least 1,500 calories' worth of jogging, brisk walking, or other vigorous activity each week had a 25 percent lower death rate during the study period than those who expended less than 1,500 calories a week.

The more active the men were, the longer they were likely to live—even the men with bad habits like smoking and drinking. Researchers agreed that exercise increased their longevity because it reduced the risk of heart disease.[5]

But you aren't ready to take on the challenge of vigorous exercise? Most of us aren't. Don't worry; moderate exercise will do just fine.

THE FINISH-LINE POWER
OF MODERATE EXERCISE

The *John Hopkins Medical Letter* boldly proclaimed: "Exercise is by far the most effective prescription for healthy aging."[6] If you are going to beat the aging clock, exercise is absolutely essential.

Maybe you have been promising yourself for years to get up off the couch and start moving. You are just looking for a great way to get started. Well, moderate walking for exercise has proven effective in increasing longevity for millions.

Two studies, the Honolulu Heart Program and a twin study in Finland, confirm that exercise, walking in particular, has very positive effects in terms of longevity.[7] Even when risk factors were removed, the protective effects of exercise were still amazing. The study revealed that walking two miles a day can reduce your risk of dying by 50 percent. The twin study in Finland revealed that conditioning exercises reduce the risk of dying by 43 percent.[8]

The evidence supporting a link between how much you exercise and how long you will live is absolutely overwhelming.

WHAT EXERCISE CAN DO FOR YOU

The US Surgeon General's report on physical activity calls for thirty minutes of moderate exercise a day. When you exercise enough to break a sweat, and you do it regularly, your body will realize loads of life-extending—and even life-saving—benefits. Let's take a look at some.

Preventing heart disease

In an American Heart Association report Dr. Roy Shephard of the University of Toronto and Gary Balady of Boston University Medical Center performed an analysis of a hundred different studies. They found that all researchers uniformly agree that regular moderate exercise can lower blood pressure, reduce cholesterol, reduce the overall risk of heart disease, and prevent dangerous blood clots.

Exercise helps those who have already suffered a heart attack too. In addition, the benefits of exercise can be seen on a daily basis. Individuals have lower blood pressure on the days they exercise than on the days when they don't exercise.[9]

Just in case you are not convinced that physical laziness is killing us, here is a statistic that may shock you. As many as 250,000 deaths each year in the United States are due, at least in part, to our sedentary lifestyle. Astonishingly that is almost one-fourth of all deaths in the United States![10]

Those who do not exercise are twice as likely to die suddenly from heart attacks.[11]

Building up brain cells

Believe it or not, some researchers think that jogging and other moderate exercises may have the power to stimulate your production of brain cells. Where once it was thought that brain cells could not reproduce, that theory has become passé. Researchers have now proven otherwise through experiments in which mice that were allowed to choose exercise grew new brain cells while sedentary, bored mice did not.

Fred Cage, a neurologist at the Salk Institute in La Jolla, California, sought to discover what kind of exercise was most important to the production of brain cells. Researchers kept a control group of mice stuck in ordinary cages while a second "runner" group were allowed to run as they pleased on an exercise wheel. Two other groups were designated as the swimmers. One group of swimmers had to learn a maze, while the other mice were put in a shallow pool every day to swim. The runners grew more brain cells than the sedentary mice and even the swimmers.[12]

Gage couldn't say for sure that the runner mice with more brain cells were actually smarter because of them. But he says it is reasonable to assume that they might be smarter because the new brain cell growth took place in the part of the brain that is linked to learning and memory.[13]

Reducing risk of stroke

A brisk walk, bicycling, or gardening for just one hour a day may also cut your risk of having a stroke in half. Stroke is the third leading cause of death in the United States after heart disease and cancer. Researchers from Boston said that moderate exercise can reduce important stroke risk factors such as high blood pressure, obesity, and diabetes. In addition, it can also reduce the tendency for the blood to clot, further reducing the risk of stroke.[14]

An ongoing study that was started in 1962 has tracked the health of 11,130 men who graduated from Harvard between 1916 and 1950. The results are extremely interesting:

+ Men who expended 2,000 to 3,000 calories through exercise a week were 46 percent less likely to suffer a stroke.

+ Oddly, men who exercised vigorously and often, enough to burn up 3,000 calories a week, did not reduce their risk of stroke further. As a matter of fact, the risk for these men was actually higher than it was for moderate exercisers but comparable to those who burned only 1,000 to 2,000 calories a week.[15]

When it comes to reducing your risk for stroke, moderation is the key. In addition to reducing the risk for stroke, moderate exercise also has a greater effect at lowering blood pressure than vigorous exercise.[16]

Preventing other diseases

> ✦ The ways in which exercise will help to strengthen your body against diseases are impressive. Let's look at a few more: Exercise improves blood flow and lowers cholesterol levels.
>
> ✦ Exercise lowers the risk of certain cancers (colon, prostate, endometrium, and breast).
>
> ✦ Exercise prevents or controls type 2 diabetes.
>
> ✦ Exercise staves off osteoporosis by increasing bone density.

In addition, regular exercise will just make you feel better. It gives you more energy and promotes self-confidence. Exercise also releases endorphins into your bloodstream, which gives you an overall sense of well-being.

What Kind of Exercise Should I Get?

It is pretty difficult to refute the powerful, life-extending benefits of exercise. Check with your doctor or health care practitioner to see what kind of exercise is best for you. You should never begin any exercise program without first seeing your doctor.

Aerobic training

Aerobic exercises are those exercises that are rhythmical and repetitious in nature, and they are good for large-muscle groups. Aerobic exercises include walking, jogging, cross-country skiing, stair climbing, swimming, basketball, rowing, and skating. Make sure your aerobic exercises give both your arms and legs a good workout.

If you plan to start walking, here are some pointers:

+ Walk on a sidewalk whenever possible.

+ If a sidewalk is not available, walk against traffic.

+ Cross only at intersections, and use crosswalks.

+ Make eye contact with drivers.

+ At night wear light-colored clothing, preferably with reflectors, and carry a flashlight.

+ Stay out of drivers' blind spot, which is next to the rear of the car on either side.

Shoes are very important, and walking shoes are different than other exercise shoes. Here is what to look for in a walking shoe:

+ Avoid inside seams that cause injuries.

+ A half-inch heel will prevent overstretching of your Achilles tendon.

+ Your walking shoes should have a wider heel than other athletic shoes and should fit snugly.

+ If you have flat feet, remove the inside foam arch support.

+ Be sure there is a half-inch space between your big toe and the front of your shoe.

+ Be sure your footwear has soft upper material.

Resistance training

Resistance training, or training with weights, can increase muscular strength and endurance in both men and women. Don't think that you are too old for weightlifting. Even if you are elderly, resistance training can still produce the most dramatic results for you.

Working with weights is especially beneficial for building bone density. "Lifting weights and other resistance training can be even more important than other forms of exercise in fighting osteoporosis and obesity," said Dr. Thomas Perls of the Harvard Medical School's Division on Aging.[17]

You don't need to pump iron with heavy barbells every day, however. Get a set with which you can do eight to fifteen repetitions without stopping. By doing eight to ten different exercises two days a week, you can realize an enormous improvement.

If you are younger than fifty, work your major muscle groups two to three days a week with weight loads that permit eight to twelve repetitions. Older patients should exercise with weight loads that allow ten to fifteen repetitions.[18]

Flexibility training

Flexibility training increases the elasticity of joints while reducing the risk of injuries. Start with a modest flexibility program two to three times a week that includes range-of-motion exercises to stretch all major muscle and tendon groups.

Establish short-term goals for yourself that are both realistic and reachable. And once again, remember that you should never begin any exercise program without first seeing your doctor or health care practitioner.

SOME FINAL POINTERS

Let me finish with some final pointers that can help you move from a sedentary lifestyle to a more active one. To begin with, just move more. Becoming an active person can involve thousands of tiny little choices you make throughout your day to move around. Here are a few:

- Start taking the steps instead of the elevator.

- Walk to the kitchen to get your own drink of water instead of asking someone to bring one out.

- Walk to the mailbox instead of stopping at it when you pull into your driveway.

- Walk to the corner store to get the paper instead of having it delivered.

- Instead of sitting down to watch another night of television, go miniature golfing.

- Take a walk along the beach.

- Take ballroom dancing lessons.

- Choose an exercise you find enjoyable and do it.

- Plant some flowers in the dead spot in your front yard and spend a few evenings a week digging around in the dirt.

- Walk next door to check on your neighbor instead of calling on the telephone.

The list is endless, and you probably can come up with many more ideas than I have listed here. What is important is that you make these hundreds of little choices to be more active and then follow through with them. These tiny decisions will act like little stones paving a road to an entirely new attitude, renewed health and energy, and ultimately to a longer life. Decide today to get moving!

Chapter 10

LIFESTYLE AND LONGEVITY: OVERCOMING HABITS THAT STEAL YEARS

I've had eighteen straight whiskies,
I think that's the record... [1]

—LAST WORDS OF POET DYLAN THOMAS

THE FIRST TIME I met Jennifer (name has been changed), she was being rushed to the emergency room on a stretcher. A doctor was pumping air into her lungs to save her life. It took the better part of an hour to get tubes and IVs in place to medicate her and get her vital signs under control. After the commotion was over and all the infusions and tubes typical in intensive care units were in place, Jennifer, just a teenager at the time, was rendered grave but stable.

Jennifer had a collapsed left lung due to fractured ribs following a head-on collision. She had been returning home from a party where her boyfriend drank too much before he got behind the wheel. She survived because she was wearing a seat belt, but the impact of the collision had cracked her rib cage against the restraining action of the belt.

The number one cause of death in teenagers is automobile accidents. I'm all for teaching our kids about safety and responsible driving, but we must also teach them about the perils of a destructive lifestyle.

Dr. Lester Breslow, a California public health specialist, found that seven specific unwholesome health habits can shorten life or increase disability. He studied the lives and habits of seven thousand men and women in the Oakland section of California's Alameda County for more than three decades. His discoveries come as little surprise.

The more poor habits these people practiced, the greater their chances were of dying in ten years. And even when their bad habits did not lead to an early death, these individuals increased their risk of suffering debilitating physical and medical limitations that stole away much of their enjoyment of latter years.[2]

Four of the unhealthy practices that emerged from the study are easy to guess:

- Drinking too much alcohol

- Smoking

- Being overweight

- Not getting enough exercise

However, other unhealthy habits are somewhat less expected. They include the following:

- Sleeping too little or too much (more or less than seven to eight hours a night)

- Eating between meals

- Not eating breakfast[3]

Dr. Breslow does not claim that these last three are as bad as excessive smoking and drinking. Instead, he believes that they indicate a chaotic lifestyle, and those who do them probably pay inadequate attention to their overall health and well-being.

The most impressive good habit was regularity. Regularity in your living habits is a strong indicator of good health and potential longevity.[4]

Research from the Karlsruhe Institute of Technology supports these claims. Participants completed surveys and medical and fitness tests a total of four times between 1992 and 2010. Many factors were considered, including the participants' fitness level, eating habits, and smoking habits. Each of these factors were shown to have an effect on the participants' health for the duration of the study: eighteen years.[5]

WEALTHY, HEALTHY, AND WISE?

Another lifestyle indicator for longevity is income level. Wealthy people live longer than those with more modest incomes. In fact, those at the higher end of the income scale live a full five to ten years longer than the rest of us. Higher income earners more commonly avoid risk factors such as smoking, excessive drinking, and overeating. They also tend to pay better attention to good nutrition and eat less fat. Those with more cash also tend to join health clubs more often and appear to be more committed to regular exercise. The wealthy also get better medical care, drive safer cars, and live in safer neighborhoods.

But wealth certainly doesn't buy longevity. What it buys, however, is good health care, better education, and healthier lifestyle choices.[6] The direct correlation between longevity and education is largely due to lifestyle choices based on better options.

But if you don't have a job that pays you a lot of money, don't worry. You are not doomed to suffer a premature death. I have listed below some lifestyle choices that can be made by everyone, rich and poor alike. These are all behaviors that anyone can follow, no matter how much money you make.

- You don't have to join an expensive spa; just take an evening walk.

- You don't have to hire a personal physician; just get regular checkups.

- You don't have to eat the most expensive cuts of meat; just be sure that what you eat is lean.

Healthy lifestyle choices are not the property of the wealthy and well educated. They can be yours too. All you have to do is choose them!

WHY WOMEN LIVE LONGER

In chapter 3 I briefly mentioned that women live longer than men, and I gave some examples. Appendix B shows the 2013 average life expectancy of men and women from the United States, Switzerland, Japan, and Sweden—and the differences. Have you ever wondered why women live longer? Although we have already noted that genetic factors play a part, some experts believe that lifestyle choices may also hold a key. For example, Mormon men who are well known for their healthy lifestyles and lack of personal vices tend to live as long as Mormon women.[7]

For the general population, however, here are the lifestyle factors that tend to shorten a man's life:[8]

- Men take more risks and traditionally hold more dangerous jobs.

- Men tend to hold the most dangerous positions in the military.

- Men tend to visit doctors less often than women.

+ Men are more likely to be heavy drinkers and smokers.

+ Men tend to eat less healthy diets.

So if you are a man who believes that real men don't eat quiche, perhaps you should rethink your gender bias. Why not give quiche a try? You may feel a little better and live a lot longer if you do.

A MATTER OF CHOICE

The Carter Center sponsored a conference called "Closing the Gap," attended by 120 of American's foremost experts on health, including several Nobel laureates. Discussions revealed that we as individuals have a much greater role to play in our health and longevity than do hospitals, medicines, and high technology. Two-thirds of our physical ailments and premature deaths are caused by our own deliberate choices of lifestyle, and they can be delayed or prevented with proper habits.[9]

Here is a summary of these experts' advice:

+ Do not smoke.

+ Maintain recommended body weight.

+ Exercise regularly.

+ Minimize consumption of foods high in cholesterol and saturated fats, sugar, and salt.

+ Don't drink excessively, and never drive when drinking.

+ Wear seat belts.

+ Remove handguns from the home.

+ Have regular medical exams, including blood
    pressure tests.[10]

These are simple lifestyle principles, but nationwide studies show that few people observe them. This neglect costs Americans about a third of our useful lives.[11] How you live and what you do without a doubt impacts the length of your life.

BAD HABITS AND
PREMATURE DEATHS

I was once invited to a show at which the famous comedian George Burns was to be interviewed. Mr. Burns was ninety-nine years old at the time. The dialogue between the interviewer and Mr. Burns went something like this:

"George, tell us, do you smoke a lot?"

"Do I smoke? The only time I'm not smoking is when I'm asleep."

"Is it true that you also have a drinking habit?"

"Well, you tell me. I drink about a liter of liquor a day."

"Do you engage in any type of exercise?"

"Never."

"Well, what does your doctor say about that?"

"I don't know what he would say. He's already dead."

The audience nearly burst their sides laughing. George Burns certainly was an exception to the principles of longevity. He was gifted with supergenes and an immunological combat force capable of resisting twelve hours of cigar smoke and a liter of liquor a day. A rare individual can smoke and drink and live to ninety-nine, but honestly, do you consider yourself to be one of them? Mr. Burns got away with his poor lifestyle choices and bad habits. Most people do not.

Bad habits and poor lifestyle choices are drastically cutting short our lives. A recent issue of the *Journal of the American*

Medical Association reported on the causes of premature deaths. Its findings are not surprising:

+ The number one cause of death in America is tobacco, which is blamed for more than 400,000 fatalities a year. In fact, thirty-five-year-olds who smoke cigarettes have already reduced their life expectancy by more than fifteen years.

+ The second cause of premature death is improper diet, causing 300,000 deaths each year.

+ The third cause of early death is alcohol, the deadly force behind 100,000 deaths per year. Many of these deaths are due to drunken driving accidents.[12]

The sad conclusion is that our lifestyle choices are leading to shortened life spans and untimely death. Barring accidents and some illnesses, the decision to live long and well lies with us. We pave a long, healthy road that stretches out before us with our choices, decisions, and lifestyle habits. Or conversely, we chop off precious minutes, hours, days, and years through our bad choices and unhealthy decisions.

IS IT TIME FOR A CHANGE?

Whether it is smoking, not exercising, eating too much sugar, or any other negative longevity-stealing lifestyle habit, it is time to make some changes. Perhaps you have tried to overcome certain habits again and again with very little success. Don't give up. Your life, especially the years at the end of your life, may be at stake.

According to John C. Norcross, professor of psychology

at the University of Scranton in Pennsylvania, and author of *Changing for Good* (Avon Books, 1995), change is a process for which you must be ready.[13] Norcross says that change is not as simple as some might suppose. He insists that individuals pass through what he calls "states of change" in the course of modifying their negative behaviors:[14]

1. *Precontemplation.* In this state, you are basically in denial. You aren't even thinking about change or considering that you need to change. At this point you must educate yourself and become convinced of your need to change.

2. *Contemplation.* At this state you have acknowledged your problem, but you aren't ready to fix it. Self-analysis can help. You must be willing to take a good hard look at the pros and cons of making the change.

3. *Preparation.* At this point you have decided that you need to change. Begin making small advances toward your goal. Purchase walking shoes if you are going to begin to walk every day. Throw away your ashtrays if you are going to stop smoking.

4. *Action.* Now you are actively putting your decision to change into action. Your new lifestyle has feet. According to Norcross, you are most at risk of falling back into your old behaviors at this state. Look for some support structures, such as encouraging friends. Throw out the cookies or cigarettes that might tempt you. Write yourself encouraging notes and stick them to your bathroom mirror and refrigerator.

5. *Maintenance*. Now you must stick with it. In addition, keep reinforcing the action state to prevent a relapse into old behaviors.

WHAT DO YOU BELIEVE?

Yosuke Chikamoto, PhD, a behavior psychologist at Stanford University in Palo Alto, California, says it is important to understand what beliefs you are holding on to that might be affecting your behavior.[15] Do you hang on to outdated notions that research theories are overblown? That the American diet is basically healthy? That you had an aunt who smoked and lived to be ninety, which cancels out all of the findings of medical research?

It is important to take a good, hard look at what you believe. Afterward you must confront yourself, and you must confront your giant—your Goliath who stands at the entrance of your personal promised land, taunting you, defeating you, and threatening to keep you from reaching your potential.

CONFRONT YOUR GIANTS

What's your giant, your Goliath? You cannot seize your victory until you confront what defeats you. What is it about you that makes it impossible for you to surmount your hurdles, whether they be harmful personal habits or well-worn paths of defeat?

There is great strength in admitting a weakness. Most of us have at least one Achilles' heel. Those who are successful get there by understanding their weaknesses and vulnerabilities and dealing with themselves accordingly.

Motivational speaker Zig Ziglar spoke about a friend who learned to handle his personal giant of pornography:

> I have a friend who became addicted to pornography and has broken the habit. Recognizing that weakness,

he is careful not to have even the slightest exposure to
anything of a pornographic nature. If he's in a place
where the television set is on and there's suggestive language or behavior that is of a lustful or seductive nature,
he immediately leaves the scene. That's smart.[16]

Another major key to confronting your Goliath is discipline. The great violinist Isaac Stern, who was instrumental
in preserving Carnegie Hall, was asked, "Is talent born?" The
question was in reference to an outstanding performance.
He responded, "Yes, talent is born, but musicians are made."
Becoming a great musician involves a vast amount of discipline,
hard work, and talent. No matter how great the talent, unless
an individual is personally disciplined, much of the potential
will remain just that—potential.[17]

Ziglar said, "Tie discipline to commitment, and it becomes
an irreversible decision that you will do today what most
people won't, so you can have tomorrow what most people
can't."[18] I believe that says it all.

You may be thinking, "That's great. When you have bootstraps to pull yourself up with, you can always succeed. But
what if you've tried and tried and discovered you have no
bootstraps? Then what?"

Help is still available. Let me explain.

YOU CAN FIND HELP

The Bible says truth makes you free. (See John 8:32.) If you
consider that negative habits and behaviors are actually personal bondages, then finding freedom becomes an important
factor. Truth is not often easy to accept—especially the truth
about yourself. It takes a strong desire for freedom to overcome the denial and self-deception that keep you locked into
lifestyles formed by negative behaviors and harmful habits.

But you can find the strength to approach difficult truths about yourself and to find freedom through faith in God. Faith is a powerful force, a force greater than any other in the entire universe. Faith is also a force that you can tap into at any moment of lack or need.

You do not have to face the power of addictive behaviors alone. At this very moment you can ask God for help, and He will not turn you away. The Bible says, "Ask, and it will be given to you; seek, and you will find; knock, and it will be opened to you" (Luke 11:9, MEV). If you are facing the power of a seemingly insurmountable habit or personal weakness, don't face it alone. Confront your Goliath armed with faith in God and an understanding that He loves you with a love that is beyond your ability to even comprehend. God Himself will help you fight the battles in your life.

Chapter 11

SETTING YOUR ATTITUDE
FOR LONGEVITY

You can't help getting older,
but you don't have to get old.[1]

—GEORGE BURNS

OFTEN A DIAGNOSIS shouts at you the minute you lay your eyes on a patient. I saw Peter (name has been changed) as he was on his way to the surgical suite. He had the typical signs and symptoms of an acute abdomen, an event that seriously endangers a patient's life, with a surgical procedure the only possibility of saving him. I instantly assessed that we were in for a complicated encounter. Although Peter was only thirty years old, he was more than 150 pounds overweight, his breathing was compromised, and—with a ruptured gallbladder and a gigantic liver cyst—he was in tremendous pain.

Heavy patients are not only risky to operate on, but they also pose a high level of difficulty. Peter's waist circumference was threatening to us all. As we began to prepare him for surgery, Lupita Leon, a nurse who has been there for us through thick and thin, in the most stressful situations, diligently prepared the operating room as she has done for so many years.

The removal of the gallbladder was difficult, and the liver cyst was extremely challenging. There were moments when we thought Peter was not going to leave the surgical suite alive.

The few hours we spent operating seemed like a year, and the stress we experienced in those moments was horrendous. But Lupita has been through many of such events and has always maintained a cheerful attitude that breaks the pressure of even the darkest of moments.

I have often wondered how Lupita has survived so many years through so many challenging surgeries and maintained her sanity. The greatest wonder about her is that she seems to be frozen in time. She shows no signs of the difficult years of work in her appearance. When Lupita is in the operating room, everything seems to be just perfect: anesthesiologists find every tool at their fingertips, and the surgical team members receive whatever they need before they ask. Lupita is always ahead of the game. Scarcely a word comes from her peaceful and pleasant face, but when she speaks, her words have significance.

Fortunately Peter's outcome was successful, but at the end of the procedure we were all physically and emotionally drained. The surgical team was heavy with the stress of the procedure, and we silently reflected that Peter's life had been spared only because it was not God's time for him to die.

Lupita, noticing the dark cloud that seemed to be descending on us, decided to come to our rescue. It was nearing lunchtime, and she looked at the clock, smiled, and said, "Did somebody say McDonald's?"

Lupita's attitude has helped to keep her, and the rest of us, young. Interestingly her wonderful outlook on life seems to actually be signaling her body not to age.

Attitude is a powerful force. And your own attitude is powerful enough to increase the length and quality of your life or to diminish it.

AN ATTITUDE THAT SAYS YOUTH

Having the right attitude is clinically proven to extend your days on earth. As a matter of fact, researchers say that much of aging is in the mind.

Many researchers are realizing that your prospects for good health and a long life are remarkably dependent on your attitudes—your psychological, emotional, and philosophical outlook on life. Your attitudes cause emotional reactions in your body that strongly and very directly impact your immune system, circulatory system, and even your risk of accidents.[2]

For example, in 1973 Dr. Grossarth-Maticek tested thousands of elderly citizens of Heidelberg, Germany, for attitude. He measured habitual feelings of pleasure and well-being. Twenty-one years later he compared the individual's tests scores with their overall health records. The results were utterly astonishing. The three hundred individuals who had scored highest in terms of attitude and well-being were thirty times more likely to be alive and well twenty-one years later than the two hundred lowest scorers.[3]

An individual's attitude proved to be a much more effective predictor of future health and longevity than all other factors such as genetics, lifestyle, smoking, and diet![4]

This suggests that improving your attitude can have a greater long-term impact on your health than improving your diet, exercising, quitting smoking, or losing weight. Think of the benefits in terms of extended good health and increased longevity you can have if you address all of your risk factors.

YOUR ATTITUDE AND RETIREMENT

It is absolutely true that, although we all age, we do not age at the same rate. Some enjoy great health and vitality for far more years than others. And, of course, some live far longer with many more productive years than others. It is also a well-known fact that many individuals age more quickly and experience more ill health after they retire if they do not continue to pursue meaningful activities. Who hasn't heard of the poor aunt or great-uncle whose health seemed to fail right after entering a nursing home? Do such persons adopt fatalistic attitudes that undermine their futures?

It might interest you to know why Western countries have a sixty-five-year-old mandatory retirement age. When Bismarck was chancellor of Germany in the 1870s, he noticed that virtually all of his powerful enemies were men who were sixty-five years old or older. He persuaded the German legislature to pass legislation making sixty-five the mandatory age for retirement. It had nothing to do with a decline in mental capacity. As a matter of fact, it was their wisdom, experience, power, and organization that made these men such a threat. For some strange reason, other countries in Europe followed Germany's decision, and the policy regarding retirement was eventually adopted in America.[5]

YOU ARE AS
YOUNG AS YOUR HOPE

Our culture encourages individuals to begin winding down their expectations when they have reached their peak of intellect, wisdom, contacts, power, experience, organization, and influence. Douglas MacArthur spoke powerfully about attitude and aging in his farewell address to the cadets at West Point:

> Whatever your years, there is in every being's heart the love of wonder, the undaunted challenge of events and the unfailing childlike feel for "what next" on the job and in the game of life. You're as young as your faith, as

old as your doubts; as young as your self-confidence, as old as your fear; as young as your hope, as old as your desperation. In the central place of your heart, there is a recording chamber. So long as it receives messages of beauty, hope, cheer and courage, so long are you young.[6]

Many researchers believe that certain attitudes can contribute to longevity, healing, extended vitality and good health. Optimism, reducing anxiety, learning to deal with anger, responding creatively to change, looking forward to life, and integrating new things and fresh ideas into your life can all impact longevity.

Let's take a closer look at some of these life-extending attitudes.

FOREVER HOPEFUL

Have you ever met a person who seemed happy, hopeful, and at peace no matter what devastating blows life threw at them? We all have. Such individuals actually live longer, stay younger, and seem to enjoy the ride much more than the rest of us.

Hope, according to the dictionary, is "a feeling that what one desires will happen. It's expectation, anticipation, optimism; the ground for expecting something desired."[7]

Zig Ziglar spoke about hope also. He said, "A hopeful man is someone who would take his last dollar and buy a money belt."[8]

Martin Buxbaum summed it up beautifully: "No matter what the difficulties, the trials, the disappointments, those who have risen to the top never lost hope. Hope gives us the promise of something good, despite the odds, something we can attain. Hope sets the mind in a positive vein, gives us something to look forward to and patience to wait. Hope is a heart-warming blend of desire, expectation, patience and joy. It is an emotional medicine, indispensable to the soul."[9]

THE POWER OF EXPECTATION

Hope and expectation go together like a hand and glove. Your hopeful expectations are filled with power to open doors and to pave a pathway to your desired expectation. But your negative expectations hold a darker power in your life, even when it comes to aging. Do you expect to get old, feeble, and ill? If so, you probably will. Many experts believe that there is great power in your expectations. Much of aging is in the mind, and debunking old, depressing stereotypes about aging can have a powerful effect.

By deprogramming ourselves from the conditioning we have received over the years—twenty-five thousand hours in childhood alone—we can mentally slow down the aging process. A Yale news article claims that a good attitude can extend life more than some healthy habits.[10]

According to Bernie S. Siegel, MD, one of the best ways to make something happen is to predict it.[11] Most medical professionals generally accept that a "placebo effect" can actually impact the outcome of an illness. In other words, if a patient believes he is taking a miracle drug, or if she believes that she is able to be cured, that individual will draw on internal forces and occasionally make it happen. Therefore your attitude about your own longevity will have a tremendous effect.

DISEASE-BEATING ATTITUDES

Changing your attitude can change your life. I have heard it said that William James wrote, "The greatest revolution of our generation is the discovery that human beings by changing the inner attitude of their minds, can change the outer aspects of their lives."[12] Years of experience have taught me that cancer and, indeed, nearly all other diseases are psychosomatic. This may sound strange to people accustomed to thinking that psychosomatic ailments are not truly "real," but believe me, they are.

Each one of us has the power to deal positively with the dark emotions that attempt to plague our minds. Arnold Hutschnecker, author of *The Will to Live* wrote, "Depression is a partial surrender to death, and it seems that cancer is desperation at the cellular level."[13] We are under emotional pressure constantly. There are crises and wars everywhere. How can we avoid the stress that anguish, fear, and depression cause?

Our bodies react to the attitudes with which we confront the events, problems, challenges, experiences, memories, and expectations of our lives. In other words, how we respond to the negative events in our lives will show up in our bodies. Researchers are just discovering how depression, pessimism, excitement, and optimism directly affect our immune systems. Interestingly, in the second century, physician and philosopher Galen postulated that depressed men and women fell prey to cancer easier than those of a happier, sanguine temperament.

Evidence exists that housewives who feel useless get cancer 54 percent more often than the general population. Amazingly a 157 percent higher incidence of cancer strikes these women as compared to their counterparts who work outside of the home. But wives and mothers who feel they make a vital contribution because they are an irreplaceable team member in the family have a lower incidence of cancer.[14]

SETTING YOUR SAILS ON AN OCEAN OF HOPE

A strong dose of hope will impact everything about you. It will affect your health, your lifestyle choices, the quality of your relationships, and how long you live. Hope is not an attitude that some possess and others do not. Those with a great deal of hope choose it. They decide to choose hope over hopelessness, optimism over despair, and faith instead of defeat.

As you set your own mind toward hope, you will be setting the sails on the course of your life. Hope will take you where negative emotions can never go. With hope, optimism, and courage you can learn to sail above the waves that crash against your life, and you can find true peace and genuine faith.

Close your eyes. How do you see yourself at age one hundred? Will you be found riding a bicycle while enjoying the countryside, as Jeanne Calment did at age one hundred? If you expect to die alone, depressed, and ill, you probably will. But if you determine to build a new outlook of hope for the future, it certainly can't hurt you, and it may release you from a lifetime of negative attitudes and their consequences.

Set hope as one of your life goals. No matter how negative you have been in the past, you can reset your sails right now. When you choose to be hopeful despite negative circumstances, you strengthen your sense of optimism and increase your ability to hope.

Make a plan right now to do something spectacular on your one hundredth birthday. If it is throwing a party, plan the menu and the music. Find other unusual, truly creative ways to build and express your sense of optimism and hope about the future.

EMBRACING CHANGE AND LEARNING TO GO WITH THE FLOW

Another attitude to sail on is flexibility. Researchers name flexibility among the attitudes that strongly contribute to longevity. Other attitudes that contribute include these:

+ Responding creatively to change

+ Reducing anxiety

+ Turning into your creative and inventive resources

+ Being very adaptable

+ Integrating new things and ideas into your life

+ Looking forward to life

You will notice that all of the attitudes listed above involve coping with change in positive ways. Perhaps the old proverb is true: If you can't bend, you will eventually break. We all might as well accept that the only constant in our lives is change.

Learning and growing experiences have a physiological impact on your body. A group of elderly people who learned to play the organ showed an increased blood level of human growth hormone after their learning experience. Researchers have linked this raised hormone level with enhanced well-being.[15]

FLEXIBILITY AND SURVIVORS

THE TELEVISION series *Survivor* has us all thinking about what it takes to be a survivor. Psychologist Al Siebert studied the personalities of a few survivors of a military unit that had been virtually wiped out in Korea. These individuals displayed attitude qualities that made them unique and, no doubt, carried them through. Those who beat the odds against them were tough but more patient than the doctor had expected. Their response to mistakes was usually to joke about them instead of getting angry.

As Siebert continued to study survivors, he discovered that a primary characteristic of beating the odds is an unusual degree of flexibility. The most prominent characteristic of a survivor is a complexity of character, a union of many opposites. These individuals are serious and playful, tough and gentle, logical and intuitive, hardworking and lazy, shy and aggressive, introspective and outgoing. These paradoxical people don't easily fit into neat categories, and their complex character traits cause them to be far more flexible than other people.[16]

According to Siebert, it is possible to learn to be a survivor. Here is a list of survivor traits:[17]

+ Enjoying work for its own sake, like a happy child

+ An ability to become so absorbed in your work that you lose track of external events, time, and all of your worries, often whistling, humming, or talking to yourself

+ A willingness to look foolish, make mistakes, and laugh at yourself

+ An open-minded acceptance of criticism about yourself

+ An active imagination, daydreams, mental play, and conversations with yourself

+ Empathy for other people

+ Able to see patterns and relationships in organizations or equipment

+ Good timing, especially when speaking or taking an original action

+ The ability to spot early clues about future developments and take appropriate action

+ Cooperative nonconformity; refusing to be controlled by improper laws or social standards, yet choosing to abide by them most of the time for the sake of others unless attempting to change them

+ Being comfortable in complex, confusing situations that others find bewildering and frightening

+ Keeping a positive outlook and confidence in adversity

+ The ability to absorb new, unexpected, or unpleasant experiences and be changed by them

+ The ability to convert what others consider accidents or misfortunes into something useful

+ A feeling of getting smarter and enjoying life more as you get older

It is important to see yourself not merely as a secretary or boss or mother. In other words, don't see yourself in terms of a role. Don't think of yourself as a collection of habits, such as, "I'm a smoker," "I'm a worrier," or "I'm a go-getter." Think of yourself as a living being, created in the image of God Himself, an individual who is ever changing, constantly taking on new challenges and continually growing.

When you lose your ability to grow, change, try new things, and enjoy fresh, exciting experiences, you will begin to die. A growing, breathing, evolving, living being will continue to thrive—even in old age.

The Bible speaks about staying fresh in your mind and heart. The psalmist wrote in Psalm 92:12–14:

> The righteous man will flourish like the palm tree,
> He will grow like a cedar in Lebanon.
> Planted in the house of the LORD,
> They will flourish in the courts of our God.

They will still yield fruit in old age;
They shall be full of sap and very green.

—NAS

A tree that is full of sap and very green is one that is filled with vitality, life, and youth. These scriptures suggest that God's will for us is that we feel better, look younger, and live longer! No matter what our age, we can be a fruitful tree, full of fresh ideas, new dreams, much hope, and great expectations. That is God's desire for us.

Make a decision to embrace change, look for new challenges, and dream about your future. Decide now never to grow stale and tired, and most importantly—never grow old!

Chapter 12

LAUGHTER AND LONGEVITY

*I would not live forever, because we should not
live forever, because if we were supposed to live forever, then we would live forever, but we cannot live forever, which is why I would not live forever.*[1]

—ANSWER GIVEN BY MISS ALABAMA
IN THE 1994 MISS USA CONTEST WHEN ASKED,
"IF YOU COULD LIVE FOREVER,
WOULD YOU AND WHY?"

A MAN WITH CANCER is informed by his primary physician that he will be dead in an hour. He runs to the window, looks up at the sky, and says, "God, save me!" Out of the blue comes a wonderful, melodious voice saying, "Don't worry, My son. I will save you." The man climbs back into bed filled with faith, hope, and peace.

In the meantime his physician has left his bedside and called an oncologist. The oncologist walks into the room and says, "If I operate in an hour, I can save you."

"No, thanks," replies the man. "God will save me."

Then a radiation therapist walks into the room and says, "If you let me start treating you immediately, I believe I can save you."

"No, thanks," the man answers. "God will save me."

Finally a nutritional therapist enters the room and says to the man, "I believe I can save you if we get started with a nutritional program right away."

"No, thanks," says the man. "God will save me."

After the hour is up, the man dies. When he gets to heaven, he walks up to God and says, "What happened? You said that You would save me, but I died, and here I am."

God answers, "Well, I sent you an oncologist, a radiation therapist, and a nutritional therapist! What more did you want?"

Sometimes health and healing come from unexpected places—like laughter, for instance. Humor has a power to lift you above life's circumstances where you can find health, healing, and release from pain, stress, and other deadly, longevity-robbing emotions. A good sense of humor can add years to your life.

Julie dramatically discovered the amazing power of laughter. She came to Dr. Bernie Siegel's organization, ECP, because of her blindness, which was the result of diabetes. Once, while out to dinner at a restaurant, her family and friends sat her down in a chair, and she, presuming the table was in front of her, inched her chair forward. She kept inching and inching forward, and ended up across the room. The entire restaurant watched in silence, not knowing how to respond. Finally, she bumped into another table, where the people asked, "Would you like to join us?"

As soon as Julie realized what had happened, she began to laugh uncontrollably. And when she did so, the entire restaurant exploded with laughter.

Julie has since regained her sight—truly a healing miracle. When speaking about her blindness, she says, "Blindness taught me to see." Julie now works as a therapist at Dr. Siegel's organization.[2]

Julie was truly unique. Her infectious gift of humor allowed her to transcend a disability that would have hurled others into a pit of depression and despair. Laughter is a powerful weapon in your arsenal against aging. Let's take a closer look.

BOOST YOUR IMMUNE SYSTEM
WITH LAUGHTER

In a series of studies at Loma Linda University in California, researcher Lee Berk discovered that watching a comedy video can strengthen your immune system in very measurable ways. Just as stressful emotions such as grief and anger can suppress your immune system, positive emotions such as laughter can have the opposite effect. When a group of people were tested after watching a comedy video, they all measured higher in immune system functions.[3]

"Silliness is very serious stuff," said Dr. Berk, one of America's foremost researchers on humor and health.[4] Berk's studies revealed statistically significant reductions in cortisol levels along with increases in antibodies that fight infection, cytokines that regulate immune function, and natural killer cells that seek out and destroy viral and tumor cells.[5]

A good belly laugh boosts the body's immune system and reduces hormones that cause stress. A positive state of mind helps keep healthy people well and helps the sick recover.[6]

"There is a lot of medicinal value to laughter," said psychologist Don Powell, founder and president of the Farmington Hills, Michigan–based American Institute for Prevention Medicine. His organization incorporates laughter seminars into corporate presentations on stress management. "Laughter is a natural sensation that has positive effects both mentally and physically. It can increase circulation, stimulate digestion, and lower blood pressure. It can also reduce muscle tension," he said.[7]

Interest for research into the healing power of laughter was fueled by Norman Cousin's 1979 book, *Anatomy of an Illness*. In it he shares how he got relief from the pain of a degenerative disease by laughing his way through humorous videos.

Dr. Berk and his partner, Dr. Stanley Tan, are pioneers in the field of laughter research called *psychoneuro immunology*.

Their lab tests reveal that dramatic decreases take place in us after we chuckle our way through a funny video. Stress hormone levels, including epinephrine and dopamine, go way down after a good laugh. In addition, some of the changes to the immune system are still in your body the day following a good laugh.

Here is a list of measurable changes that take place in your body after you enjoy a good laugh:[8]

- The activity and number of natural killer cells that attack tumor cells and viruses without the help of other cells increase.

- More helper T cells that help to organize the immune system's response are activated.

- There is an increase of the antibody immunoglobulin A, which fights respiratory tract infections.

- There is more gamma interferon, a hormone that causes the immune system to turn on. Gamma interferon fights viruses and regulates cell growth.

- There are more B cells, which cluster near lymph nodes and produce antibodies against harmful microorganisms.

- There is more "complement 3," which helps antibodies pierce infected or dysfunctional cells.

LAUGHTER AT THE CELLULAR LEVEL

So then, when you laugh, this is an overview of how your body changes at the cellular level:

+ Cells that produce antibodies increase in
number.

+ Cells that combat viruses fall into formation
and get ready for battle.

All of this is the direct result of a good joke![9] No wonder comedians like George Burns live so long!

LAUGHTER, A CELLULAR CONDUCTOR

Researchers Lee Berk and Stanley Tan noted that in addition to boosting your immune system, laughter plays an interesting role in the overall harmony that your immune system needs to work at its very best. Dr. Berk was amazed by the findings, as was psychologist Paul McGhee. "It is astonishing to think that something so commonplace as laughter could manipulate significant immunological processes," McGhee said.[10]

Imagine that all the systems in your body are members of an orchestra that must perform together in harmony. One system needs to increase its volume because of a flu virus. Another system needs to play a little softer. Two systems need to blend at one particular moment to produce a special effect. Well, laughter comes into the symphony and acts as a conductor, bringing harmony and balance to all of the other performances.[11]

Tan said, "All these neuro-hormones act like an orchestra; each instrument makes a particular note. Laughter makes the entire orchestra more melodious or balanced. In other words, laughter brings a balance to all the components of the immune system."[12]

According to Berk, mirthful laughter modulates specific immune system components like the conductor of an orchestra. The conductor has the option to increase tempo and volume, rendering the music harsher, more rapid, and less harmonious. The conductor can also calm the tempo, enhance sonic integration, and make sure the body harmonizes in a healthy performance.[13] Laughter is certainly a potent force.

EVERYBODY LOVES A CLOWN

Are you a wise guy, given to telling a joke or two? Telling jokes as well as hearing them makes an impact on your body. The brain itself is affected during joke telling. Peter Derks of the College of William and Mary, Williamsburg, Virginia, says that brain wave activity physically changes when we laugh.[14] And psychologist Paul McGhee says that frequent laughter relaxes muscles, helps control pain, may lower blood pressure, and helps manage stress.[15]

LAUGHTER AND EXERCISE

Researchers have discovered that laughter and exercise trigger similar responses. Just as what happens with athletes, laughter shows increases in good hormones such as endorphins and neurotransmitters in test subjects. These individuals also show decreased levels of stress hormones, such as cortisol and adrenaline.

THE LOSS OF CHILDHOOD LAUGHTER

Children laugh about four hundred times a day, but the average adult laughs only six to eight times per day. Humor comes naturally to children. A child's inquisitive mind delights in every new discovery, and social interaction always begins with a smile. Having fun seems to be the motive behind nearly every childhood activity.[16] But as an adult, your life experiences are probably miles away from these. Does the following scenario sound like you?

You sit in a traffic jam for an hour while your car overheats and as your children wait to be picked up at day care. While you click off the minutes on your dashboard clock, thinking about missing your meeting this evening, thinking about the dinner you need to prepare and the laundry that must be done, your body sends signals to your brain that are not good for your health. Negative experiences cause your body to release increased levels of stress hormones, including cortisol, growth hormone, beta-endorphin, and prolactin. The result is that you feel stressed out. That stressed-out feeling makes your blood pressure rise and causes a host of other longevity-stealing physical reactions to take place.

The playfulness of childhood is replaced by the serious stresses of adult life. Barry Bittman, MD, says that stress is no more than a perception with measurable detrimental effects that include high blood pressure, increased blood sugar levels, and impaired immunity. "It should be no surprise that the long-term effects of ongoing stress have been proven to lead to serious illness," said Dr. Bittman.[17] We have been using laughter therapy at the Oasis of Hope Hospital for over fifty years with our patients with amazing results.

LAUGHTER AND STRESS

Stress, however, is a matter of perception. The overwhelming stress that one individual experiences when his car is scratched is not experienced at all by another individual when the same thing happens to his car.[18] Some people maintain an even keel when faced with enormous adversity, while others overreact to very slight pressures.[19]

The effects of perceived stress on your body include high blood pressure, increased blood sugar levels, and impaired immunity. Laughter has the opposite effect. Good stress, called "eustress" (*eu* in Greek means "well" or "good"), that is caused by laughter produces lower levels of stress hormones, which causes you to feel good. The physical impact on your body is very positive. You live longer and feel better when you laugh a lot. Laughter is actually a form of good stress, or stress in reverse. Having a good belly laugh is the ultimate stress buster.

Much research has shown that bad stress suppresses your immune system. Drs. Tan and Berk wanted to find out if laughter, or good stress, could act as an antidote to stress. They studied a group of average adults and found that, indeed, the group was powerfully impacted by laughter. The subjects of the studies sat through a solid hour of riotous fun as they watched videos of comedians. A control group sat quietly out of earshot. The research doctors took blood samples every ten minutes during and after the laughathon.

The researchers proved medically that laughter is a safety valve for the body—a counterbalance to tension. When we are stressed out and filled with tension, laughter causes our elevated levels of stress hormones to drop back down to normal. The result is that our immune systems are able to work more effectively.[20]

I once knew a woman who worked in one of the most stressful, demanding positions imaginable. Yet she looked at least ten to twenty years younger than she actually was. When she became stressed, she became very funny and laughed continually. Her joking and laughter were often infectious, bringing everyone around her into the fun. Her sense of humor was able to deflect the power of her stressful job off of her body. Today she continues to look younger than ever, and she continues to laugh just as often. She is a walking testimony to laughter's ability to minimize the aging effects of stress on an individual's body.

REDUCING YOUR STRESS FACTORS

Are you stressed out? You are not alone. More than 75 percent of all Americans see their lives as being too complex. Work and family stress pile on fatigue and stress-related emotions and can create a looming sense of hopelessness and futility.

The causes of stress and anger are many. Here are the top ten reasons for feeling stressed out:[21]

- ✦ Conflicts with loved ones
- ✦ Money problems
- ✦ The pace of modern life
- ✦ Working and raising a family
- ✦ Excessive noise
- ✦ Crime in the community
- ✦ Violence on TV and the movies
- ✦ Health problems
- ✦ Commuting
- ✦ Computers

Do you feel stressed out at work? Work stress is high on America's most wanted list for the stressed out among us. As a matter of fact, violence in the workplace is a growing concern for many. And why shouldn't it be? Jobs are becoming increasingly demanding, pressures to produce increase all the time, and politics in the workplace can become unbearable, even to the most placid among us.

Technology, once believed to be the savior that would relieve us of stress, simplify our lives, and bless us all with more free time, has done the opposite. Instead of more time, our clocks seem to tick faster with each technological breakthrough. Employees who are electronically monitored report anxiety, depression, exhaustion, and fear about twice as often as similar employees who are not monitored.[22]

LAUGHING AWAY STRESS

Humor is a quality of perception that enables us to experience joy even when faced with extremely stressful circumstances.[23]

Nurses who work in stressful environments that place powerful demands on them physically, mentally, emotionally, and spiritually can end up emotionally exhausted and spiritually depleted. If you feel this way at work, burnout and a caustic sense of cynicism are not far away. For nurses, chronic exposure to job stress can lead to burnout, which nurse Christine Maslach defines as "a syndrome of emotional exhaustion and cynicism that occurs frequently among individuals who do 'people work' of some kind."[24]

Because nurses are compassionate and caring people who work with those who are suffering, they are at great risk for job burnout. Nurses experience a sense of failure when their efforts are ineffective. They become angry and frustrated when patients object to their care, and they grieve when they die. Constantly experiencing such a wide range of emotions leads to stressful changes within their bodies and the hunt for something to combat the stress.

LAUGHTER, A STRESS-BUSTING TOOL

Nurse Patty Wooten says that humor can be used as a stress buster against the physical impact of job stress.[25] The experience of laughter momentarily breaks feelings of anger and fear and replaces those rancid emotions with carefree, lighthearted and hopeful moments. It is not uncommon for nurses to experience compassion fatigue, a sense that there is nothing left to give. Such feelings can occur in other strongly dependent relationships, such as caring for an elderly parent or for a disabled child. But finding humor in the midst of work, even for the emotionally weary, can replenish compassion and renew emotional energy—as in the case of Lupita Leon.

LAUGHTER, A MEDICAL TREATMENT

In 1979 Norman Cousins began treating his own life-threatening disease with laughter. But Cousins wasn't the first to prescribe laughter as a medical remedy. In the 1300s Henri de Mondeville, a professor of surgery, wrote, "Let the surgeon take care to regulate the whole regimen of the patient's life for joy and happiness, allowing his relatives and special friends to cheer him, and by having someone tell him jokes."[26]

Cousins spent the last twelve years of his life at UCLA Medical School in the Department of Behavior Medicine finding scientific proof for what Dr. Mondeville espoused in the Middle Ages. Realizing that stress created high blood pressure, muscle tension, immunosuppression, and many other negative effects on the body, Cousins sought to determine if laughter did the opposite. He proved scientifically that laughter is the perfect antidote for stress.[27]

A sense of humor allows us to perceive and appreciate the incongruities of life and provides moments of joy and delight. These positive emotions can create changes in the brain that buffer the effects of stress on the immune system. Remember my friend who laughed away her stress? Laughter provides a cathartic release, cleansing us from negative emotions and releasing tension.

HOW STRESS-PROOF ARE YOU?

Stress rolls off some people like water off a duck's back, while others seem to go looking for things to be stressed out about. Sociologist Suzanne Kobassa defined three characteristics, which she termed "hardiness factors," that cause some individuals to be more stress-proof than others: commitment, control, and challenge.[28] Have you ever thought about how well you cope with stress as compared to others around you? What defense mechanisms do you employ? Are they healthy ones, or do they tend to be unhealthy?

If you have a strong commitment to yourself and your work, if you believe that you are in control of your choices in life, and if you see change as challenging rather than threatening, then you are more likely to cope successfully with stress.[29] Many experts agree that a main ingredient to burnout is a sense of powerlessness.

Humor allows us to feel a certain sense of detachment when the heat is on. This sense of detachment, even in the very worst of circumstances, provides a feeling of control that makes it possible to cope.

When stress- and burnout-prone nurses were tested to measure their sense of control and their sense of humor, the results were amazing. Researchers were able to prove that a good sense of appropriate humor has a direct and powerful impact on a person's ability to feel a sense of control. If individuals are encouraged and guided to use humor, they can gain a sense of control over the circumstances in their lives. Although we often cannot control the events in our workplace and external worlds, we do have the ability to control how we view these events. We also have the ability to choose how we will emotionally respond to them.[30]

ANGER, STRESS, AND REPRESSED EMOTION

Tension, fear, and anger can contribute to high blood pressure, with the potential to trigger strokes or heart attacks. According to Samuel J. Mann, MD, the real culprit behind many high blood pressure readings is repressed emotion.

Emotions are powerful, yet too many people stuff explosive emotions like anger, hatred, and even rage into a closet somewhere deep inside of them. As the years go by, the closet becomes increasingly full, and the door that has been tightly closed over these emotions becomes weaker and weaker. Eventually, unable to escape through a more appropriate pathway, the power of these locked emotions undermines the entire structure. In other words, a body's health is compromised.

According to experts, when a hypertensive patient is ready to confront a painful past, the benefits not only are emotional but also improve a person's odds of living even farther into the future.[31]

The power of anger

What emotions are the opposite of laughter and fun in your life? Anger? Rage? Unforgiveness? Revenge? These are powerful emotions that will rob years from your life if you don't deal with them properly.

Anger is like burning jet fuel. It makes an individual want to explode, slam a fist into a wall, lay on their horn, or tell off a clerk. This burning fuel is ripping marriages apart and tearing up lives. Uncontrolled and mismanaged anger is the number one cause of divorce. Conflicts in personal relationships are inevitable, but handling anger is a gift that must be learned.[32]

Getting real

Although you may have carefully hidden your repressed emotions way out of sight, they are nevertheless very real, and they are probably having a much greater impact on your life than you suspect.

To begin dealing with repressed emotions, you must first confront them. You have to get real. Ask yourself what it is that triggers your angry responses and reactions that are usually way out of proportion to the reality of an event. What do you feel right before your anger explodes and you lose control? You must investigate why your reaction was so drastic.

Usually overreactions and out-of-control explosions of emotion are the result of suppressed anger from the past. Many people have a pattern of suppressing their anger until the pressures, tensions, and stress become intolerable. At this point they usually erupt like a volcano, and they find themselves doing things they later regret. Such individuals haven't learned how not to overreact.

Mismanaged anger and rage are the major causes of conflict in our personal and professional relationships. According to Leonard Ingram of the Anger Institute of Chicago, domestic abuse, road rage, workplace violence, divorce, and addiction to food, alcohol, drugs and many other harmful things are just a few examples of what happens when anger is not managed properly.[33]

The first step in controlling your anger is to stop pretending that you don't get angry. So, rule one for dealing with anger: *stop pretending.*

Coworkers, spouses, family members, and friends who deal with angry people are in line for their own kind of stress-related health risks. Learning how to diffuse an individual's anger rather than fueling it can help. Learn how to stop defending yourself and how to begin addressing the other person's anger, which is the real issue. Rule two for dealing with anger: *learn to diffuse anger.*

STOP BEING A VICTIM

Rather than being victimized by someone else's negative behaviors, here are some things you can do to understand what is coming your way and why.

You can tell the purpose of someone else's anger or other negative behaviors by the way it makes you feel when it is happening. Instead of reacting to the emotional behavior of the other person, you can ask yourself, "How is this behavior making me feel right now? What is this person—either knowingly or unknowingly—attempting to accomplish?"

1. If you feel annoyed or irritated by a person's behavior, that person may be *trying to get your attention.*

2. If you feel powerless and out of control, that person may be *trying to gain power over you and trying to control you.*

3. If you feel hurt, that person may be *seeking revenge against you.*

4. If you feel discouraged or helpless, that person may be *withdrawing from the task or situation for which he or she feels inadequate to cope.*[34]

How do you know if you have resolved your issues of anger or have merely controlled your anger by shoving it back into your internal closet? Here are a few indicators of resolved anger versus controlled anger that will, no doubt, spill over again in time.

CONTROLLED ANGER	RESOLVED ANGER
• Defensive about criticism • Blames the victim • Struggles for power • Breeds resentment • Exits persons from the system • Increases frustration and hopelessness • Demands others to get with the program	• Willing to talk about anger-causing issues • Identifies the real problem • Builds alliances • Develops self-satisfaction • Offers support • Builds trust and hope • Invites creative solutions[35]

If you are struggling with issues of anger and other unresolved emotions, get help. Start by acknowledging that you have a problem. Although it may be very difficult for you to admit and accept at first, the benefits of getting real about your situation can lengthen your life considerably. Five minutes of anger or frustration deplete the immune system for more than six hours.[36]

More importantly, if anger is a problem for you, you may be taking yourself and your life far too seriously. Why not learn to laugh again? You are not powerless in the face of your own emotions. You can set the tone and atmosphere for your own life. Sow a little laughter into others around you, and you will reap a harvest of goodwill. The experience of laughter momentarily banishes feelings of anger and fear and provides moments of feeling carefree, lighthearted, and hopeful. Laughter is the perfect antidote to dark, negative emotions.

LAUGHTER TO LIGHTEN YOUR LOAD

So many of us have carried the weight of the world on our shoulders for so many years that we have become sourpusses. We sit in a traffic jam and act as if waiting two or three minutes is the end of the world. Someone cuts in front of us, and we are ready to kill. We won't live very long if we don't learn to lighten up a little.

If you tend to take yourself and your life too seriously, it may be time to throw some extra baggage overboard and lighten your load. Take a careful look at your boat; it may already be slowly sinking. But you won't know it until it starts to take in water and you drown.

You learned to be a sourpuss; you can also learn to laugh. Humor is an acquired ability to see life's events in a light-hearted way. Here are some pointers for honing your funny bone.[37]

+ Seek out people with a special flair for seeing the funny side of a situation. Laughing is contagious.

+ Subscribe to funny literature, visit funny web-sites, and purchase joke books.

+ Learn to tell jokes. Practice being funny. Even if you bomb out on a joke, you can still get a laugh.

+ Stay in touch with your inner clown, that playful, childlike nature that we all have but perhaps fail to acknowledge due to the serious-ness of our work.

Humor can give you wings that will help you to soar above a world filled with bitterness, strife, anger, jealousy, and compe-tition. The Bible says, "All the days of the afflicted are evil, but he who is of a merry heart has a continual feast" (Prov. 15:15). Two people can experience the very same circumstances yet experience life completely differently. One feasts on the joy of life, despite his or her circumstances, and the other is weighed down by burdens that seem impossible to bear. The difference between these two points of view can be as simple as learning to laugh. Laughter is the key to a long and joyful life.

The Bible also says that laughter is like taking a prescription. "A merry heart does good, like medicine" (Prov. 17:22). This truth from the Bible is a scientific fact. Laughter, smiling, and fun cause endorphins to be released in your brain, which give you an overall sense of well-being.[38] So take the Bible prescription and laugh more often. You will add years to your life, strength to your soul, and resilience to your mind and body.

I wonder if Anna's mourners laughed as they chiseled out her headstone:

> Here lies the body of our Anna
> Done to death by a banana
> It wasn't the fruit that laid her low
> But the skin of the thing that made her go.[39]
>   —INSCRIPTION ON ANNA HOPEWELL'S
>   GRAVE IN ENOSBERG FALLS, VERMONT

Chapter 13

ALL YOU NEED IS LOVE

For love is as strong as death.

—SONG OF SOLOMON 8:6

TWO OF MY patients illustrate the dramatic power of love's impact on the physical body. An athletic, nineteen-year-old woman in love with her sport came to see me. She suffered from cancer of the small intestines. Her doctors had given up hope after a course of chemotherapy had utterly failed to halt the growth of her tumors. Medically speaking, her prognosis under these conditions was death within three to six months.

This young athlete was slated to represent her country in the upcoming Olympic games within eight months from the date she entered Oasis of Hope hospital. She shared that she came to see me because she refused to accept the prognosis of her own doctors. Under no circumstances would she be kept out of the upcoming competition.

She began her treatment with lots of faith and discipline. The results were indeed amazing. Our patients who have this kind of tumor rarely beat it. But the determination and tenacity of this girl stimulated her defenses so powerfully that they destroyed her tumor. In reality, our treatment merely served as an emotional reinforcement. We loved her, plain and simple. Our staff surrounded her with huge doses of ongoing love and support. To date, this patient is alive and healthy.[1]

The opposite occurs as well. For example, a forty-eight-year-old woman came to our cancer clinic with breast cancer after her left breast had been surgically removed. Only faint traces of her former beauty remained. Her skin was dark gray, she was bald, and her body was so emaciated that she looked as though she had been in a concentration camp.

This once lovely woman's cancer had been complicated by metastasis in the bones and lungs. Conventional therapies had failed, and her doctors had sent her home to die.

Following our nontraditional cancer treatment, she began to improve. Her hair grew back, she gained weight, and before long she looked like a new person. Although surgical mutilation had dealt her a painful blow, she had overcome it.

But sadly, once her husband saw that she was stronger, he decided to ask her for a divorce. She viewed the request as a rejection of her mutilated body. Three weeks later she experienced an explosion of new cancer tumors. Although she came back to see me, she confessed that the loss of her husband's love represented the worst kind of rejection. Life had lost all meaning for her. Her immune system crashed, and the tumors took advantage of the open door and killed her.

Love and Health

A popular song tells us that without love we are nothing. Love is certainly a powerful force—more powerful than we may have even imagined. Scientists have proven that those who have strong, loving relationships live longer and healthier lives than those who do not.

The link between love and longevity is not just heart knowledge. The power of love has been scientifically proven. A Swedish study revealed that fifty-year-old men who had gone through high levels of emotional stress alone, without the support of family or close friends, were three times more likely to die within the next seven years than those whose lives were peaceful. Other men who had undergone similarly stressful experiences but also enjoyed a great deal of emotional support from many supportive relationships in their lives had no increase in mortality.[2]

What were the stressful circumstances that were linked to an early death? They included the following:

+ Serious concerns about a family member

+ Being forced to move

+ Feelings of insecurity at work

+ Serious financial trouble

+ Being the target of a legal action[3]

Researchers concluded that experiencing stress without having strong supportive relationships may lower resistance to disease. But when you have caring individuals nearby to talk to about stressful events, emotional reactions are dramatically reduced. Therefore the loving relationships in your life help you stay healthy.[4]

DOES YOUR SPOUSE
SHOW YOU LOVE?

Does your wife give you a kiss in the morning? Does your husband put his arm around you in public? Does your spouse hold your hand at the dinner table? All of these are innocuous, sweet-but-too-sappy displays of affection, right? Wrong! Such loving signals could be saving your life.

A remarkably revealing study on love was completed in Israel by Jack Medoli and Yuri Goldbourt. The two researchers studied ten thousand men with high-risk conditions like angina pectoris, anxiety, high cholesterol, and irregular heartbeats—all ingredients for a fatal heart attack. They determined through psychological testing who would develop a heart attack and who would not. After all was said and done, the ones who had the highest incidence of heart attacks were the ones who answered no to the question "Does your wife show you her love?"[5]

According to Leo Buscaglia, insurance companies have discovered that men who leave for work in the morning with a kiss from their wives have fewer car accidents and will live an average of five years longer than those who leave without a kiss.[6] If it wasn't for the fact that insurance companies are in the business of evaluating risk to increase their revenues, I don't know if I would believe it. But there it is, simple and romantically scientific!

These revolutionary findings of the twentieth century were well known centuries ago to the Hebrew people. Biblical proverbs extol the value of loving relationships:[7]

> Rejoice with the wife of thy youth.
> —PROVERBS 5:18, KJV

> He who finds a wife finds a good thing.
> —PROVERBS 18:22

LOVE YOUR PARENTS

Do you maintain a close, loving relationship with your elderly parents? If you do, it might be extending their lives.

A thirteen-year-long study tracked health changes and deaths of 220 elderly parents to determine if intergenerational bonds impact longevity. Researchers found that the elderly tend to live longer if they have loving relationships that provide practical aid, such as people who drive them to the doctor's office or help them at home. The surprising conclusion: loving ties with middle-aged kids do more to lengthen life than any other support.[8]

Haitao Wang of the University of Southern California surveyed parents and children every three years, taking account of health, age, marital status, and education. Here are some of his findings:

+ Parents who felt close to their children were least likely to become depressed or disabled.

+ Parents who received any practical help from kids were 20 percent less likely to die than those getting none.

+ Even after taking into account practical support from offspring, those who felt above-average closeness with their children were 40 percent less likely to die over a thirteen-year period than those who felt below average in closeness with their kids.[9]

THE BIOCHEMISTRY OF LOVE

Although love research is in its infancy, studies are beginning to confirm its positive effects. The Menninger Foundation of Topeka, Kansas, found that people who were in love have lower levels of lactic acid in the bloodstream, which causes them to feel less tired. These individuals also have higher levels of endorphins, which cause them to feel more euphoric and less sensitive to pain. Their white corpuscles respond better to infection, and they catch fewer colds.[10]

In 1982 Harvard psychologists David McClelland and Carol Tishnit discovered that even films about love increase levels of immunoglobin A in saliva, the first line of defense against colds and other viral diseases. Although the increase of immunoglobin A lasted less than an hour, it could have been prolonged by having the subjects think about moments in their lives when someone loved them. If we love, we are happy, and those around us make up a part of our positive world and don't wear down our defenses.

THIS IS YOUR BRAIN IN LOVE

Do you ever wonder what physically happens in your brain when you fall in love? If you are in love, your hypothalamus tells your heart to beat faster, your powers of concentration to wane, and your thoughts to remain fixed on Mr. or Miss Right. The hypothalamus is the area of your brain that contains a lot of connections with the associative areas of your cortex (your gray cells). It is the part of the brain that controls your perception of pain and hunger, your emotions and feelings (such as fear, anger, sadness, and love) and your biological rhythms and sexual feelings. Your hypothalamus is the manager of your emotions and feelings.

When you fall in love, your hypothalamus secretes a chemical compound called phenylethyalamine (PEA). As the PEA level increases in your blood, your brain is stimulated and produces endorphines. Endorphines, as we mentioned earlier, have almost the same effects on your brain as morphine. We actually become high on love, or euphoric on a chemical level over the person on whom we have set our affections.

What happens when Mr. Right doesn't call? What happens when your favorite girl breaks up with you? Since the endorphines act as morphine, you actually become addicted to them. When the phone doesn't ring, your body suddenly stops producing endorphines, and you experience withdrawal symptoms. You feel depressed, sad, and even angry.

This is lovelessness on a purely biophysical level. But love, hate, and rejection are much more than simply biophysical phenomena. They are matters of the spirit and of the heart. And the forces connected with the heart and the spirit are the most powerful forces in the human person. Love appears to be the most important power within us. Without love a baby will not thrive, and it will die within a short time. It is dangerous to live without love.

THE DANGER OF LOVELESSNESS

Lovelessness is a statistically proven health risk. Divorced persons have the highest index of cardiovascular disease, pneumonia, high blood pressure, cancer, and even fatal accidents. Did you know that divorce causes more stress than imprisonment? The amount of couples splitting for irreconcilable differences is staggering. This plague of lovelessness is creating a society of resentful, depressed adults and children who either hate themselves because they blame themselves for their parents' divorce, or they hate their parents for abandoning them.

The power of negative emotions such as depression, unhappiness, and hate is enormous. History revolves around their dominance, especially hate. Hate leads to war, destruction, and death. There is only one other emotion comparable but more powerful than hate: love.

The Bible teaches us to love our enemies. Jesus Christ said, "But I say to you, love your enemies, bless those who curse you, do good to those who hate you, and pray for those who spitefully use you and persecute you" (Matt. 5:44). But many of us feel that such high-minded principles could never work in today's road-rage society—and I would have to agree. In our own human love the assaults that assail us daily make it impossible for us to love everyone as Christ taught. The only way that we can even begin to approach living our lives with outstretched hearts, extended in love to all, is to walk in the power of forgiveness. As Alexander Pope's popular quote says, "To err is human; to forgive, divine." Forgiveness is a divine attribute that makes love possible.

LOVE AND FORGIVENESS

Forgiveness is a choice. It may be one of the most difficult choices you will ever make, but the benefits will be worth it. Forgiving is letting go of fear, anguish, and despair and refusing to cultivate and harvest those dark emotions inside your spirit any longer. Many people have a lifetime of unresolved offenses circulating through their minds and causing new stress with each recall, says Dr. Bernie Siegel. Confronting these offenses and letting go of them involves honestly facing your own part of the problem and forgiving yourself as well as the others you have resented and feared. If you don't forgive, you become like your enemy.[11]

Forgiveness is tough, dangerous, and exciting, according to Zig Ziglar.[12] It is tough because our human nature resists it, and it is dangerous because it forces us to take responsibility for our future. Forgiveness is also exciting because it frees us to become our best selves.[13]

When you forgive someone else for his or her offenses, you receive your own life back. When you harbor hatred, resentment, and anger, you are in bondage to the person who has offended you. But forgiveness cuts the cord and releases you. Now the onus is on the offender. You have passed the test, and in so doing, you have passed the test along to your offender. Whether he passes his part of the test is not your concern. You are now able to move on to your future, free from the emotional chains that kept you anchored to the past.

If you hold bitterness, resentment, or anger toward another person, you might not deliberately wish the other person ill. But if something bad happened to him or her, you wouldn't necessarily lose sleep over it either.[14] If you feel this way, then you haven't forgiven. If anything good happens to the other person, your resentment is kindled anew.[15] This is nothing less than a passive way of getting revenge. One great authority on stress, Hans Selye, says that revenge is the most destructive emotion and that gratitude is the healthiest.[16]

One of the most important keys to forgiveness is to correct any offenses immediately. When you have done something wrong and offended someone, you can go back immediately, ask for forgiveness, and explain the situation. In our stress-filled society, we all offend. But if you immediately go back and gain pardon when you have offended someone, you will be able to handle your emotions much better. Your stress level will go down, and your immune system will respond much better.

It is never too late for forgiveness, no matter what you have done. You can always go back and clean up the mess. Sometimes we expend three or four times the energy by not swallowing our pride and saying we are sorry. Many times our biggest problem is the fact that we were right. Well, the Bible tells that we should forgive those who have transgressed against us. So even when we are right, we need to go and say, "You know, I had a problem with you. I felt this—I felt that. I want to be at peace with you so that I can feel that peace with myself." It is never too late for forgiveness.

Many times we allow years to go by without mending broken bridges. The longer we wait before mending those bridges, the more difficult it is going to be. The stains of offense get stronger with time—just as it is more difficult to remove a stain from fabric if you wait too long. But if you clean it up immediately, it is removed very easily. But it is never too late.

We have patients who hadn't spoken with their children for fifteen years, but when faced with a life-threatening disease, they were finally able to open up. Let's not wait until problems become that large. Let's clean our messes immediately and become much happier people in the process.

A FORGIVENESS SELF-TEST

Take a moment to take stock of your own heart. Do you hold grudges toward people from your past? Do the little things, or big things, these individuals did come up in your mind occasionally or often? If so, then you need to make a choice to forgive.

If possible, write these people a letter and tell them you have forgiven them. But don't minimize your responsibility either. Ask them to forgive you for any part you played in the offense and also for holding a grudge toward them.

Some people may respond very well and restore the breach that was between you. Others may act as though you were the bad guy and they were faultless. It doesn't matter. Now the test belongs to them. You don't even have to be there to grade it. Just let their emotions remain their own, and let their responses remain their own as well. Now you are free.

FINDING FREEDOM
THROUGH FORGIVENESS

When King David sinned, he prayed a prayer that is recorded in the Book of Psalms. He told God, "Against You, You only, have I sinned" (Ps. 51:4, MEV). This may have been a bit of an overstatement, but it makes a point. All sin is committed against God. Nevertheless, God is a heavenly Father who is full of forgiveness. Before you can be completely free, you must ask God to forgive you. He will. Christ died on a cross in order to offer forgiveness to the entire world. You can receive that forgiveness by directing a prayer to Him. Why not try it?

If you have asked God to forgive you, you have become truly cleansed. No guilt can condemn you. The blood of Christ was shed as a great price so that your guilt could be washed clean.

Now you need to do one last thing. You need to forgive

yourself. If the God of the entire universe doesn't hold your sin against you, then who are you to do so? He is much greater than you. So what are you waiting for? No matter what you have done, let it go. You are truly free!

THE PRICE OF LOVE

Death was the price of Christ's love for you. He loves you so much that He died to wash away your guilt and set you free. Determine to follow in His wonderful footsteps, choosing to love those around you, even those who have greatly offended you. Not only will you reap a harvest of goodwill and friendship, but the benefits of unpacking your emotional baggage could also lengthen your life by considerable years.

THE GOLDEN RULE

Love is so important and powerful that Christ summarized nine commandments into one: "Love your neighbor as you love yourself." The Golden Rule, "Do unto others as you would have them do unto you," is based on Christ's summary.

Yes, all we need is love, just as John Lennon and others have sung. But why is there so little of it? My brother-in-law, Joel Ordaz, an independent minister, believes there are so many problems in the world precisely because we love our neighbors *as* we love ourselves!

It is certainly a contradicting perspective, but let's examine how we love ourselves. We love junk food, alcoholic beverages, and smoking. Love to some is never having to exercise. Our love affair with quarreling, fighting, and hating is at an all-time high. If this is how we love, then it is no wonder our backs are breaking from carrying around so much emotional baggage. Our neighbors certainly don't need this kind of love.

Self-esteem in every culture is vital to the preservation of good health, both physical and mental. Narcissists only love their own looks, but individuals who love or esteem themselves accept themselves as imperfect beings. Once you and your defects are comfortable with each other, you are more likely to be happy in this world. Those who are at peace with themselves and others will enjoy a longer and better life. This healthy love of self, or self-esteem, includes accepting responsibility for the health of your body, soul, and spirit. This is the kind of "yourself" love your neighbor needs. Even with our emotional baggage and human imperfections, love is still the answer.

PART III

THERE IS A FOUNTAIN

Chapter 14

SUCCESSFUL AGING

All flesh is as grass, and all the glory of
man as the flower of grass. The grass with-
ereth, and the flower thereof falleth away.

—1 PETER 1:24, KJV

I N A PELTING rain of ticker tape, streamers, and shredded computer paper, seventy-seven-year-old astronaut and statesman John H. Glenn Jr. paraded through the streets of New York City in a hero's celebration of his second history-making space flight. Thirty-six years earlier astronaut Glenn had received a similar tribute after being the first American to orbit the earth.

As the seventy-seven-year-old space legend orbited the earth in the shuttle *Discovery* with six other crew members, the inspired eyes of the world gazed into the silent heavens once more to watch. In a world woefully short of true heroes, we all took genuine pride at the courage, boldness, and dignity of this man.

And a true hero he was. Glenn received the Distinguished Flying Cross on six occasions, and he held the Air Medal with eighteen clusters for his service during World War II and Korea. His many other accolades include the Navy Unity Commendation for service in Korea, the Asiatic-Pacific Campaign Medal, the American Campaign Medal, the World War II Victory Medal, the China Service Medal, the National

Defense Service Medal, the Korean Service Medal, the United Nations Service Medal, the Korean Presidential Unit Citation, the Navy's Astronaut Wings, the Marine Corps' new insignia (which is an astronaut medal) and the NASA Distinguished Service Medal.[1]

But Glenn's medals of honor are not just tokens from a glorious past. Though he fought two wars and fought the heavens to gain entrance into space, his battles as a valiant fighter did not end until he fought and won one last victory. Having broken through space barriers into new vistas for science as a young man, as a seventy-seven-year-old astronaut he blasted through outdated attitudes erected against the elderly. Glenn's victory against prejudice may have been his greatest act of heroism.

Just as the world looked on with pride and wonder during his first victory in space, our sense of wonder and humble appreciation of the significance of his second journey overwhelmed us once again. John Glenn is a true American legend.

No book about longevity would be complete without addressing the issues of aging that we all must eventually face. I like the term *successful aging* because it gives us back the power to win. Even if we enjoy significant longevity, we will all grow older—it is inevitable. But we do not have to fear growing older, and we do not have to be defined by the prejudice and stereotypes that surround aging. Let's take a look at successful aging.

THE PROMISED LAND

As we prepare to enter each new season in our lives, we stand at a vista of opportunity, promotion, change, and uncertainty. As with a youngster becoming a teenager or a teenager entering adulthood, when we begin to move into the winter months of our lives, we enter a new land understanding little about its possibilities and its promise. Arriving at its border does not mean that we have entered. And entering it does not mean we have conquered its obstacles and mastered its possibilities. Our lives will take us to this season—it is inevitable. But we are the ones who must enter, conquer, and gain mastery over the new territory to which time has brought us.

Conquering Giants

The ancient Hebrews discovered that at the border of their Promised Land were giants that need to be conquered. If you are to embrace the winter season of your life, if you are to age successfully, you will discover how those ancient Hebrews felt. You will face your own set of giants.

The first giant you must face is prejudice. Prejudices regarding aging must be conquered. Society is filled with out-dated stereotypes about the winter years of one's life. But the first battlefield where this giant must be spotted, captured, and conquered is not in society at large. This giant must first be defeated in you!

Some consider old age to be a biological, lethal disease. Arlie Hochschild, in *The Unexpected Community*, refers to the elderly as society's "death lepers" because they, for the first time in history, are those most likely to die.[2]

But age is little more than the experience of time, and time, the experience of change. Each new season of development is launched and maintained through a biological code encrypted in our genes. These orders tell a baby's midsection to grow longer and his mind to form words. In our winter season this code commands our brown hair to change to gray, our tight skin to sag, and our sharp eyes to grow dim. It is possible for our internal clocks to send the wrong messages, however. An eleven-year-old victim of progeria[3] dies of old age. Some individuals become psychologically old at age thirty following a major trauma, and other individuals remain psychologically young at age seventy.[4]

How you think about your own experience of aging can be spoon-fed to you by others, or it can be formed by you through careful, deliberate consideration.

SO, WHO'S OLD?

In general, our own age determines whom we consider to be an old person. When we are teenagers, anyone over twenty-one seems old. When we are thirty, forty seems old, and at age sixty, we feel compassion for the oldsters who are in their eighties. Many young-feeling individuals receive a shocking membership invitation to the AARP at age fifty, which can feel like a wake-up call or a personal invitation to a midlife crisis.

Much of what we think about as old is not real—it is just old thinking. As noted earlier, we live in the power of our expectations. As Job said, "The thing I greatly feared has come upon me" (Job 3:25). If we expect our bones to creak, they probably will. But they don't necessarily have to.

The legal definition of elderly would probably be sixty-five years of age or older, which is when Americans can begin to receive full Social Security benefits.

WHEN ARE WE OLD?

In a poll in which Americans were asked what they considered the optimum retirement age, the average answer was fifty years old. However, when the same people were asked at what age they considered a person to be old, the average answer was seventy-three years of age.

So what happens during the twenty years or so between retirement and old age? Many of us just shift from full-time work to part-time employment. Some of us do volunteer work. At one time people continued working until they died. Now we retire and live as many years not working as we were employed.[5]

"So then, when are we old?" questioned Jimmy Carter in his book *The Virtues of Aging.* "The correct answer is that each of us is old when we think we are—when we accept an attitude of dormancy, dependence on others, a substantial limitation on our physical and mental activity, and restrictions on the number of other people with whom we interact. As I know from experience, this is not tied very closely to how many years we've lived."[6]

DEBUNKING THE MYTHS

Chances are you may think of the most elderly members of our population as all either playing mah-jongg in Palm Springs while bragging about their children or sitting in a dilapidated farmhouse shivering under a tattered blanket covered with drifting snow while eating TV dinners. Or does the picture of a roomful of drooling, drugged, and wheelchair-bound, head-bobbing, gray-headed seniors parked in front of a television set staring blankly at daytime soap operas in a nursing home come to mind?

Contrary to popular opinion, the elderly are neither smoking away at mah-jongg tables in Palm Springs nor staring with hollow faces at nursing home floors. Most of our stereotypes about the elderly are not very accurate. Let's take a look at the statistics and get a clearer picture of the elderly among us.

Most elderly individuals are neither filthy rich nor dirt poor. Households with families headed by persons sixty-five or older reported a median income in 2013 of $51,486. The median income of older persons in 2013 was $29,327 for men and $16,301 for women. About 6 percent of family households with an elderly head had incomes of less than $15,000 and 70 percent had $35,000 or more.[7] How does that compare to the national average? For 2013 the median income level for the nation's households was $51,939.[8] So you can see the income figures for the elderly roughly parallel those of the entire population.

The average value of homes owned by elderly folks during this same period was $150,000, compared to a median home value of $160,000 for all homeowners. About 65 percent of these same homeowners owned their homes free and clear.[9]

There were 26.8 million households headed by older persons in 2013; of these, 81 percent were owners and 19 percent renters. The median family income of older homeowners was $34,500. The median family income of older renters was $17,300.[10]

Persons sixty-five years or older numbered 44.7 million in 2013. They represented 14.1 percent of the US population, which is about one in every seven Americans. The elderly population is growing, and that trend is expected to continue for decades to come. The number of older Americans increased by 8.8 million (24.7 percent) since 1990, compared to a 6.8 percent increase for the under-sixty-five population.[11]

There were 25.1 million older women and 19.6 million older men in 2013. This is a sex ratio of 128 women for every 100 men. The sex ratio increased with age with a ratio of 195.9 women for every 100 men for those age eighty-five and older.[12]

The number of elderly Americans is expected to dramatically increase in the coming years; it is already growing significantly as baby boomers reach sixty-five years of age. By 2040 it is estimated that there will be 82 million older persons, which is more than twice the number in 2000. About 14 percent of the population was sixty-five or older in 2013, but that number is expected to rise to 21.7 percent by 2040.[13]

The nursing home myth

Most of the elderly are not vegetating in nursing homes. Only 1.5 million seniors, or 3.4 percent of seniors, live in nursing homes or other institutional settings. These figures increase as the years march on; 10 percent of those who are eighty-five or older live in nursing homes.[14] Most seniors never live in nursing homes.

The majority of seniors lived with their spouse according to 2013 census figures. Fifty-seven percent of those not in nursing homes lived with their spouse. Seventy-two percent of older men and 46 percent of older women lived with their spouse. These numbers go down with age; 32 percent of women over the age of seventy-five live with their spouse.[15]

About 28 percent of seniors lived alone; These singles represented 35 percent of senior women and 19 percent of senior men. These figures increase as time goes on, as you might well imagine. Among women seventy-five years of age and older, 46 percent live alone.[16]

Retirement states?

Most seniors work hard all of their lives, live meagerly, and retire in Florida, where 90 percent of the state's population consists of blue-haired drivers who jam up the highways—unless, of course, they find their way to Arizona instead. Right?

That notion is a little exaggerated—except perhaps the point about drivers, which might be argued by some. More than half of the population of those who were sixty-five years and older lived in thirteen states in 2013: California, Florida, Texas, New York, Pennsylvania, Ohio, Illinois, Michigan, North Carolina, New Jersey, Georgia, Virginia, and Arizona. California is at the top of the list with 4.8 million individuals over the age of sixty-five. Florida and Texas are next, with approximately 3 million each.[17]

Florida had the highest percentage of seniors, with seniors

constituting slightly more than 18 percent of Florida's population. The next highest were Maine and West Virginia, each with approximately 17 percent.[18]

THE AGING BABY-BOOMER GENERATION

America's 78-million-member baby-boomer generation is aging rapidly. The hippie generation is now between fifty-two and seventy years old. What can they expect, and what can the country as a whole expect as this huge population glut of post–World War II, Benjamin Spock babies moves into its autumn and winter years?

Financially the baby boomers have done very well; known as having "financial exceptionalism," the baby boomers quadrupled their net worth since the late 1980s by benefiting from the economic growth and stability during their prime earning years.[19]

Many baby boomers are in the midst of what generations ahead of them are painfully aware of. By the time adults reach their midforties, heart disease, the nation's number one killer, begins to make its mark.

But baby boomers will always be somewhat different than all other Americans. This generation will always be more individualistic. Having grown up during political tumult and financial prosperity, baby boomers will probably always feel somewhat suspicious of authority and economically optimistic. The younger generation, known as Generation X, does not tend to share the optimism. They report feeling that they can't quite make ends meet.[20]

Even though baby boomers now run America, they continue to be less happy with the status quo, just as they were as teenagers and young adults. Baby boomers are also pessimistic about foreign affairs.

Financially baby boomers are heavy users of credit cards and loans. Education continues to be a major focus for baby boomers.

They are more likely to own computers, make long-distance phone calls, discipline a child, and get up before 6:00 a.m.[21]

Baby boomers will probably always enjoy the sense of financial security they have grown up with. Because many baby-boomer women have spent their lives working, many dual-income households will also become two-pension households. Older women on their own will enjoy greater economic security than their mothers knew.[22]

Baby boomers will enter their twilight years continuing to love granola, to enjoy walking, to feel selfish about leisure time, and to spend money somewhat carelessly. Don't look for this group of seniors to go out and purchase rockers. The only rocking these seniors will be involved in will doubtless be rock and roll.

THE GRAYING OF A NATION

The attention that baby boomers have experienced as consumers all of their lives will continue to follow them. Americans over sixty-five years of age already outnumber teenagers. And those sixty-five-year-olds today have not aged as quickly as generations before them. Most are well and leading full, vigorous lives. So you can expect the attitudes about seniors to be changing in the near future. The baby-boomer generation that spearheaded social change in the 1960s and 1970s will remain true to form. By virtue of sheer numbers of seniors America will change. There is little doubt of it. This large group will think for itself, have greater financial means and influence, and continue to hold its own strong opinions. Whereas America seemed preoccupied with youth when baby boomers were young, its preoccupation will turn silver, along with its boomers.

The Coming Centenarians

As we saw earlier, one of the greatest changes that America can expect in its future is the birth of an entirely new strata of society: the centenarians. Many of today's robust seniors, who once could have expected to live no longer than their eighties or nineties, can now expect to live well into their centenarian years.

Recently the number of people over the age of eighty-five grew more rapidly than the overall population. The fastest-growing group of all, however, is those over one hundred. In 1956 there were 2,500 centenarians. In 2000 there was an amazing 268,000![23]

Chances are good that if you are looking down the road toward your twilight years, you may one day find yourself among this burgeoning group of one-hundred-year-olders. Are you burning up your strength like a sprinter, or have you begun to look at your own finish line with the mind-set of a long distance runner?

The Times They Are a'Changing

The nation is changing, demographics are changing, our life expectancies are changing, and for many of us who are beginning to age, our bodies are changing as well. In the years ahead the nation will certainly look much different. In addition, the average American today has fewer children than his or her parents did.[24] What will all of these changes look like for the future? What do all these changes suggest for us as individuals? What can we expect? How should we respond?

Whether we know it or not, these changes in longevity and retirement habits place new responsibilities on us as individuals. Northern farmers know well what late summer means. It doesn't mean swimming, vacations, shopping for school clothes, or making last-minute decisions about moving and employment. For farmers from colder climates, the late summer through early fall is a time when productivity and fruitfulness are at their peak. This is the time when farmers begin to prepare for winter.

Chances are, if you are a baby boomer, your fruitfulness is also at or nearing its peak in terms of health and income. One thing we must do nowadays is to prepare for long, drawn-out illness near the end of life. In the past, medical care was designed to cure serious diseases, but with extended life spans come chronic ailments and diseases such as arteriosclerosis, osteoporosis, and Alzheimer's disease. Diseases that were at one time fatal, such as heart disease and kidney disease, can now be treated successfully, sometimes for years, with pacemakers, bypasses, dialysis machines, and even transplants. These medical procedures can help us to live normal lives and even weather the storms of once-fatal or debilitating diseases.[25]

So how do we prepare for our longer winter?

PREPARING FOR WINTER

Old-time northern farmers employed a kind of wisdom that helped them succeed and build America into the prosperous country that it has become. These agrarians purchased a little almanac that helped them predict what kind of winter they could expect so that they could get ready.

Interestingly Jesus Christ alluded to this kind of farm wisdom when instructing the leaders of His day. He said, "Whenever you see a cloud rising out of the west, immediately you say, 'A shower is coming'; and so it is. And when you see the south wind blow, you say, 'There will be hot weather'; and there is" (Luke 12:54–55).

Is the winter season of your life approaching? Will it be a long, harsh winter or a long, mild one? How far in the distant future is it? How long will it endure? Are you expecting to live into your seventies, your eighties? Have you considered what your future will be like if you become a member of the dramatically increasing numbers of centenarians?

At the moment you may well feel that you are far too young to begin preparing for your winter season. But it is never too soon to begin to prepare physically, mentally, emotionally, and financially.

Preparing for future good health

You can prepare your body physically by developing good, healthy lifestyle habits that will pave a road to future good health, no matter what your age. The foundation of health that you establish in your body actually begins in childhood. But it is never too late to start. What you eat today will make a difference in your health tomorrow. How much you exercise will also matter. Good medical care and good lifestyle habits, such as not smoking or drinking, will make an enormous difference tomorrow in how you feel and look.

We are a fast-food generation that lives for the moment. Because we don't experience the consequences instantly, we really believe that we have escaped the consequences of eating a diet loaded with fats and heavy carbohydrates or living a sedentary life. But how we cheat our bodies in our youth will have to be repaid in old age, through broken health, disease, or early death. Youth is health's credit line that must be repaid in old age. So, how heavily overdrawn are you? If you audit your own health ledger today, you won't receive an overdraft notice tomorrow.

Keeping your mental edge

I also encourage you to formulate a plan for maintaining your mental youth. In a well-known study researchers discovered that older nuns who played mentally stimulating games, worked on mentally stimulating puzzles and other challenges, and found other ways to keep learning and growing mentally displayed fewer symptoms of senility than individuals who quit challenging their minds.

What courses do you plan to take when you retire? What academic degrees do you plan to pursue? In what ways are you continuing to stimulate your brain today? Do you work the *New York Times* crossword puzzle on Sundays? Do you continue to stretch your mind, or have you quit growing intellectually?

Although memory loss is associated with old age, it doesn't have to happen to you. A long-term study at Washington University School of Medicine in St. Louis suggests that senility is not an inevitable part of aging. "Our findings support the idea that you can age successfully without the neuropathological changes associated with dementia," said John C. Morris, MD, associate professor of neurology.[26]

Recent findings at the University of Kentucky suggest a link between senility and small strokes. These strokes could actually be so slight as to go unnoticed. The study was based on autopsies of 102 nuns, half of whom had the brain lesions characteristic of Alzheimer's. Of those who had also suffered strokes, 93 percent had symptoms of Alzheimer's: memory loss and dementia. But 53 percent of those nuns who had the brain lesions and didn't suffer a stroke had shown none of the telltale debilities.

If strokes trigger Alzheimer's, then controlling the disease could actually be as simple as lowering your blood pressure, exercising, and quitting smoking—all relatively easy behavior changes that improve cardiovascular health.[27]

Preparing for your emotional future

What can you do to prepare your mind now for your years of retirement? What plans do you have for your mental future? Many of us consider our financial futures, which is extremely important. But as a doctor and scientist, I would encourage you to consider also your emotional and psychological future as well.

Jimmy Carter, in his book *The Virtues of Aging*, suggests, "We should consider life as expanding, not contracting."[28] Carter, who is now ninety-one, also said when he was in his seventies:

> A person my age now has the remaining potential that only a much younger person had just a few decades ago. We not only have longer to live, but in some ways each year now equals several years in olden times. We are exposed to fifteen times as much knowledge as Aristotle was; many of us travel as much in a year as Marco Polo did in a lifetime. In effect, as far as knowledge and observations are concerned, our life experiences encompass the equivalent of a thousand years in older generations. Our number of years have increased by 50 percent, but our functional years have grown by 1,000 percent.[29]

Anyone visiting a nursing home can quickly see that the average older person now watches television for about forty-three hours a week. With the vistas of opportunity available to us and the promise of longevity to grant us future dreams also comes the responsibility to lead, lend, and love. We must lead those who are younger and lend to the world our knowledge, insight, and wisdom, and we must love, for this is the greatest commandment.

We can be like the woman who personifies wisdom in the Book of Proverbs. She was prepared for the winter season of her life, and therefore she greeted it without fear. "She has no fear of winter for her household, for she has made warm clothes for all of them" (Prov. 31:21, TLB). If we prepare for the winter of our lives, then our winter years hold the hopeful promise of becoming the very best time of all.

Chapter 15

CROSSING THE BRIDGE

Life is a bridge. Cross over it,
but build no house on it.

—INDIAN PROVERB

PARTIALLY HOISTED SAILS gently flapped in the warm breeze as seamen and crew boarded an ancient vessel. Shielding his eyes from an unusually bright winter sun, the captain announced that winds blowing softly from the south signaled safety for the long Mediterranean voyage from Jerusalem to ancient Rome. Sailing in the first century could easily prove to be tricky business, especially during the winter months.

On the final leg of their pilgrimage these ancient travelers chose to sail as closely to the shores of the island of Crete as possible. But not long into their journey the skies turned black as a powerful storm swept across the open sea. The ancient mariners, together with the pilgrims, struggled hard to keep control of the ship as giant waves tossed the wooden vessel every which way, dashing it against great walls of water. Fighting sheets of rain and water, the seamen threw overboard all cargo and supplies.

The storm was too large and too fierce to oppose. Soon the terrified crew quickly realized that maintaining control was impossible, so they threw overboard the ship's tackle and handed over the ship to the power of the angry gale. Now the dark power of the fierce wind controlled their fate, driving the ship to parts unknown.

In the terror of days on the stormy sea one of the pilgrims shouted that he had seen a vision. They would live, but the boat would be lost. Before long the boat began to break apart, but mercifully land was spotted as well. As the raging storm began to subside, those aboard who could swim jumped into the water and went ahead of the others. Bobbing on broken pieces of wood, the rest followed. True to the prophetic vision, the vessel was destroyed. But the weary pilgrims washed ashore on a strange but beautiful island.[1]

YOU ARE A PILGRIM

I recite this story as a parable. Whether we realize it or not, each one of us is making a pilgrimage. And one day each one of us is destined to meet a storm whose power is far greater than our own. This storm will sweep down upon my life, and it will sweep down upon yours as well. So strong will be the force of its wind that we may initially throw off all the baggage of our lives that had previously encumbered us. If the winds pick up, under their power we may even begin to throw off the things that would have allowed us to bring our vessels back to safety.

One day, although we may spend our lives attempting to deny it, fight it, defend against it, and defeat it, a dark cloud will cover us, and the power of its wind will drive our destinies. When it does, we will have no ability to escape. It will take us from what we know to another place that we haven't known. Who we are and what we have become on our journeys will wash up on the shore of another place. But the vessel that carried us for many faithful years will not make it. It will be destroyed in this final sail.

As surely as our pilgrimage of life began at birth, our lives will end under the dark clouds of death. So why do we live our lives searching for a mythical fountain of youth? Many of us desire to escape the power of aging, but most of us also long to escape a much more fearsome force: the power of death. As I mentioned in the opening chapters of this book, we long to live forever young. Therefore I'd like to end this discussion of our search for the fountain of youth with a bold proclamation: There is a Fountain! Let me tell you about it.

ETERNITY WITHIN

Before I begin, let me take you through a little exercise to help you to see yourself in a different dimension. It is designed to help you to better understand what you are and what you are not.

In your mind, picture a horse. Any picture of a horse will do, like Black Beauty or even Mr. Ed. Take a moment and examine this picture. Look at the horse. Smell it. Hear it run if you can. Now answer this question: Who is looking at the mental picture of the horse? Obviously your physical eyes are not seeing the horse. Your nose is not smelling the horse, nor are your ears hearing him. So who is seeing and smelling the horse? Who is listening to the horse run?

You are!

In fact, you are the person, the individual, the being who creates and looks at mental pictures. From a lifetime of your experiences, you know you have a mind filled with mental pictures. But you are not your mind or the mental pictures. You are a being who has the ability to create and then look at the pictures you have created.

Now get the picture of the horse back again. From what location are you viewing this mental picture? In your head? On a little movie screen in your brain? If you think about the place where the real you is located, you will realize that you have no physical location in the natural realm. You exist and are separate from the material or physical universe.

Your life is fundamentally a nonmaterial quality of existence, while the physical world is a material quantity of existence. You have a mind, and you have a body. But you are a
being. You generate ideas with the mind, and these engage the
brain to move your body. Nevertheless, you are a person, an
individual, a being.[2]

You are a spirit being with a soul who lives in a body. When
God created Adam, He blew His breath into him, and Adam
became a living being. Genesis 2:7 says, "And the LORD God
formed man of the dust of the ground, and breathed into his
nostrils the breath of life; and man became a living being." That
breath was God's own life. God created Adam's body from the
material world, but Adam's being came from God Himself.

The Bible also informs us that we were created in the image
of God. "Then God said, 'Let Us make man in Our image,
according to Our likeness; let them have dominion over the
fish of the sea, over the birds of the air, and over the cattle, over
all the earth and over every creeping thing that creeps on the
earth'" (Gen. 1:26). An image is a pattern or imprint. Since
God is a spirit being, we are spirit beings also.

The person you see when you look in the mirror each
morning is not really you. What you see is your body, which
houses the real you. The spirit/soul person inside of you is who
you really are. Just as the breath of God transcends the materials of the earth and the physical realm, so does your spirit
man transcend your physical being. Your spirit man will live
in your body for a fixed number of years. But just like the pilgrims whose lives reached beyond the life of their boat, so the
real you will live beyond the life of your body.

ETERNITY BEYOND

When Grama Alicia was ninety-four, she suffered a mild stroke
that partially paralyzed the right side of her body. Even though

her mind was intact and as sharp as ever and her ability to communicate was virtually unaffected, she felt daunted by the fact that for the first time in eight decades she was as dependent on others as when she was a child.

When family members spoke with her, she was as cheerful as always. But when we asked how she was doing, she would answer with her signature "Good, good" and then add, "I'm waiting and waiting, but it seems God has forgotten about me." Grama was happy with her life and lived full of expectation for her death. She was filled with peace, ready to cross the bridge from this life to the next. Grama waited for three years to make that final journey. In the end, she had been confined to her bed. But no space could limit the love and wisdom she radiated to us all, surely a reflection of a greater love, which comes only from above.

So what is beyond us? Where does our spirit man go when it leaves our body? What happens when we die?

The veil separating us from eternity is obscure but not completely unknown. According to a Gallup poll, 8 million people in the United States have had near-death experiences, which have allowed them a glimpse at what lies beyond.[3] This is about the size of the population of New York City. But the term "near-death" experience can be a little misleading. These experiences actually occur moments after a person has expired and before they have been revived.

As medicine becomes increasingly more sophisticated, bringing people back who have actually crossed the bridge through death is growing more and more common. Many of those who have gone through the veil and come back bring back such similar reports that it is impossible to discount them.

Death is a bridge that we must all cross over. Like the billions who have passed this way through life, we will join their ranks at the rate of approximately 130,000 a day. And in that

same day, approximately 400,000 new lives will be born.[4]
It is impossible to consider the life beyond our own without
thinking about God. The Bible says, "God is to us a God of
deliverances; and to GOD the Lord belong escapes from death"
(Ps. 68:20, NAS). Those of us who cross the bridge to eternal
life will encounter God.

In the near-death experience the spirit/soul leaves the physical body, usually after a major trauma such as an accident, illness, problems in surgery, cardiac arrest, anaphylactic shock,
coma, fever, or suicide. There are many reports from those
who have had near-death experiences.

Historians have always relied on accounts of eyewitnesses to
create accurate records of historical events. Many such eyewitness accounts of near-death experiences—running the gamut
from good to bad—are available from individuals whose lives
were dramatically changed when they visited eternity and
returned. And regardless of whether or not we believe such
accounts, the spiritual world, although unfamiliar to us, is very
real indeed.

Life on earth is a bridge that we cross to take us to eternity with God. Our walk across this bridge should be enjoyed
tremendously. But it is also a preparation of something much
better to come.

ETERNITY IN GOD

Amazingly the eyewitness accounts of such near-death experiences, although often told in nonreligious language, often parallel what the Bible says about eternity. Let's take a brief look.

Many individuals who have near-death experiences speak
of encountering light when they come near to the presence of
God. The Bible agrees with that. It says, "The King of kings
and Lord of lords, who alone has immortality, [dwells] in
unapproachable light" (1 Tim. 6:15–16).

Many individuals testify that they have encountered Jesus Christ as the Supreme Being during near-death experiences, including former atheists. Jewish individuals have said they encountered a Supreme Being they called the Messiah. The Bible says that Jesus Christ is the Son of God, the brightness of God's glory, the very image of His person, the one whom the angels worship in heaven.

> His Son, whom He has appointed heir of all things, through whom also He made the worlds; who being the brightness of His glory and the express image of His person, and upholding all things by the word of His power, when He had by Himself purged our sins, sat down at the right hand of the Majesty on high, having become so much better than the angels, as He has by inheritance obtained a more excellent name than they.... But to the Son He [God] says: "Your throne, O God, is forever and ever."
>
> —HEBREWS 1:2–4, 8

As the writer to the Hebrews says in the passage above, Christ is more than a prophet or an ancient teacher. Christ exists as God enthroned above the angels.

WHAT ABOUT ANGELS?

Those who have had near-death experiences often speak about encountering angels. The Bible speaks of them as well. Hebrews 1:13–14 says of Christ and angels, "But to which of the angels has He ever said: 'Sit at My right hand, till I make Your enemies Your footstool'? Are they not all ministering spirits sent forth to minister for those who will inherit salvation?"

Throughout the Bible, ancient men and women often saw and spoke with angels. (See Genesis 18; 19:1–22; 32:24–32; Judges 6:11–21, 13; Luke 1:5–22, 26–38; Acts 12:5–11.)

A RENEWED SENSE OF LOVE

A great percentage of those who have had near-death experiences return from them with a wonderful sense of God's love for them and for all mankind. This supernatural love of God for mankind is also written about throughout the Bible. John 3:16 says, "For God so loved the world, that he gave his only begotten Son, that whosoever believeth in him should not perish, but have everlasting life" (KJV).

EVIL SPIRITS AND HELL

Many of those who have encountered the world beyond met not only angelic spirits but evil spirits also. James 2:19 speaks of demon spirits. It says, "You believe that there is one God. You do well. Even the demons believe—and tremble!"

Hell is also mentioned in the Bible as a place that holds the dead. Revelation 20:13 says, "The sea gave up the dead who were in it, and Death and Hades delivered up the dead who were in them."

A PLACE CALLED HEAVEN

Some who have encountered death speak of going to a meadow where beautiful flowers radiated with colors they had never before seen. Some say they met loved ones who had died years earlier. Is there really a heaven? The Bible speaks of heaven when it says, "But you have come to Mount Zion and to the city of the living God, the heavenly Jerusalem, and to an innumerable company of angels" (Heb. 12:22, MEV).

THE RIVER OF LIFE

Throughout the Bible we also see mentioned a river mentioned in heaven. This river is the river of life. Revelation 22:1–5 says:

> And he showed me a pure river of water of life, clear as
> crystal, proceeding from the throne of God and of the
> Lamb. In the middle of its street, and on either side of
> the river, was the tree of life, which bore twelve fruits,
> each tree yielding its fruit every month. The leaves of
> the tree were for the healing of the nations. And there
> shall be no more curse, but the throne of God and of the
> Lamb shall be in it, and His servants shall serve Him.
> They shall see His face, and His name shall be on their
> foreheads. There shall be no night there: They need no
> lamp nor light of the sun, for the Lord God gives them
> light. And they shall reign forever and ever.

These waters that flow through heaven are called the fountain of life. Revelation 21:6 says, "I am the Alpha and the Omega, the Beginning and the End. I will give of the fountain of the water of life freely to him who thirsts."

DRINKING FROM THE FOUNTAIN

There is a fountain from which each one of us is invited to drink. Its waters give us eternal life.

During His ministry on earth Jesus Christ sat near a well and spoke to a woman who was rejected by her peers because of her many failures. He told her, "Whosoever drinketh of the water that I shall give him shall never thirst; but the water that I shall give him shall be in him a well of water springing up into everlasting life" (John 4:14, KJV).

Jesus Christ was talking about this fountain. How do we drink from it? What determines how we will spend our eternal future? Romans 6:23 says, "For the wages of sin is death; but the gift of God is eternal life through Jesus Christ our Lord" (KJV).

The Bible says that Christ paid the price of every sin on the cross. Romans 5:12 says, "Through one man [Adam] sin entered the world, and death through sin, and thus death spread to all men, because all sinned." Because Christ paid the price of sin, we can be freed from it by believing in Him. Because of Christ we can spend eternity in heaven. He is the Fountain!

Jesus told us, "I am the way, the truth, and the life. No one comes to the Father except through Me" (John 14:6). By repenting for our sins and choosing to believe in Him, we can drink from the fountain. John 5:24 says, "Verily, verily, I say unto you, He that heareth my word, and believeth on him that sent me, hath everlasting life, and shall not come into condemnation; but is passed from death unto life" (KJV).

CROSSING OVER—
A MATTER OF FAITH

For many believers science is an enemy of God—just as religion is the opiate of society according to agnostics. In my experience, science and religion are not water and oil, but are more like water and fish. I have found through science a refreshing exposition of God's work and presence. I have used quite a bit of scientific evidence in this book to entice you to take advantage of God's design and creation. Knowledge is powerful, while ignorance can be deadly.

Many agnostics and theologians reject a biblical God who allows suffering and pain and who sends people to hell. But do you believe that rejecting God will take away the pain and suffering? Remember Einstein's simple but profound statement: "The real problem is in the minds and hearts of men."

Solomon wisely said, "In the way of righteousness there is life; along that path is immortality" (Prov. 12:28, NIV). Regardless of religious inclinations, I, like most of you, believe in an immortal soul. For that reason I embrace a personal God. Without Him eternity seems dreadful and scary. But I believe that our lives have purpose and our actions have consequences, and since immortality is along the path, I choose to seek God's righteousness to reduce the risk of falling in the natural path of my treacherous mind and heart. Since this is a matter of faith, I choose God.

All we need to do to experience the evidence for God is to use our five senses. Look around and you will see that "the heavens declare the glory of God; the skies proclaim the work of his hands. Day after day they pour forth speech; night after night they reveal knowledge. They have no speech, they use no words; no sound is heard from them. Yet their voice goes out into all the earth, their words to the ends of the world" (Ps. 19:1–4, NIV).

Many agnostic astrologers, after seeing the glory of God and the work of His hands, have come to the conclusion that there is a God after all. Many have accepted that life was created, and that it is impossible for random events to have developed intelligence. But still, for most, this God is impersonal and distant. I have one more message for them and for you:

> For God so loved the world that he gave his one and only Son, that whoever believes in him shall not perish but have eternal life.
> —JOHN 3:16, NIV

I encourage you to administer responsibly your wonderfully and wondrously made body so that your life will be prolonged with quality for those possible 115 or 120 years. But more importantly, I beg you to prepare your soul for immortality, for life is merely a bridge over which we all must cross. Choose to direct your eternal future to the proper place—that place where you will live long and well, that place where you will live forever young!

Appendix A

HOW DIFFERENT NATIONS STACK UP

AUSTRIA

Life expectancy (2013)[1]

    Male: 79 years at birth (22 at age 60)
    Female: 84 years at birth (26 at age 60)

Infant mortality rate (2015)[2]

    2.1 infant deaths per live 1,000 births

FINLAND

Life expectancy (2013)[3]

    Male: 78 years at birth (22 at age 60)
    Female: 84 years at birth (26 at age 60)

Infant mortality rate (2015)[4]

    1.3 infant deaths per 1,000 live births

JAPAN

Life expectancy (2013)[5]

    Male: 80 years at birth (23 at age 60)
    Female: 87 years at birth (29 at age 60)

Infant mortality rate (2015)[6]

    .9 infant deaths per 1,000 live births

SWITZERLAND

Life expectancy (2013)[7]

Male:	81 years at birth (24 at age 60)
Female:	85 years at birth (27 at age 60)

Infant mortality rate (2015)[8]

    2.7 infant deaths per 1,000 live births

UNITED STATES

Life expectancy (2013)[9]

Male:	76 years at birth (22 at age 60)
Female:	81 years at birth (24 at age 60)

Infant mortality rate (2015)[10]

    3.6 infant deaths per 1,000 live births

Appendix B

AVERAGE LIFE EXPECTANCY OF MALES AND FEMALES IN FOUR DEVELOPED COUNTRIES IN 2013[1]

COUNTRY	MALES	FEMALES	DIFFERENCE	WHOLE POPULATION
United States	76	81	5	79
Switzerland	81	85	4	83
Sweden	80	84	4	82
Japan	80	87	7	84

NOTES

INTRODUCTION
EXPLORE YOUR POSSIBILITIES

1. A fictional account derived from facts provided by "World's Oldest Person Dies at 122," CNN, August 4, 1997, accessed January 21, 2016, www.cnn.com /WORLD/9708/04/obit.oldest/; D. Harman, "Aging: Phenomena and Theories," *Annals of the New York Academy of Sciences* 854 (November 20, 1998): 1–7; M. C. Young, ed., *Guinness Book of Records* (New York: Bantam, 1997), 11.

CHAPTER 1
IN PURSUIT OF THE FOUNTAIN OF YOUTH

1. Robert Frost, *The Poetry of Robert Frost* (New York: Henry Holt and Company Inc., 1979).
2. Dylan Thomas, *Dylan Thomas: Selected Poems*, ed. Walford Davies (London: Dent, 1974), 131–132.
3. "Juan Ponce de León, Biography," Biography.com, accessed January 21, 2016, http://www.biography.com/people/juan -ponce-de-le%C3%B3n-9444105.
4. Ibid.
5. "Fountain of Youth," Wikipedia, accessed February 22, 2016, https://en.wikipedia.org/wiki/Fountain_of_Youth.
6. N. K. Sandars, *The Epic of Gilgamesh* (Harmondsworth, England: Penguin, 1960).
7. James George Frazer, *The Golden Bough: A Study of Magic and Religion, The Magic Art and the Evolution of Kings*, 3rd ed. (London: Macmillan, 1911, 1966), 168–169.
8. Information obtained from exhibit information from a museum in China.
9. Frazer, *The Golden Bough: A Study of Magic and Religion, The Magic Art and the Evolution of Kings*, 90–91.

10. James George Frazer, *The Golden Bough: A Study on Magic and Religion, Adonis, Attis. Osiris: Studies in the History of Oriental Religion*, 3rd ed. (London: Macmillan, 1914, 1966), 3–23.

11. Peter Kelder, *Ancient Secret of the Fountain of Youth* (Gig Harbor, WA: Harbor Press Inc., 1985), accessed January 21, 2016, http://www.lib.ru/URIKOVA/KELDER /Ancient_Secret_of_the_Fountain_of_Youth-Peter _Kelder.pdf.

12. Karl Taube, *Aztec and Maya Myths* (Austin: University of Texas Press, 1993), 33–39; John Bierhosrtst, ed., "Up From the Death Land," *The Hungry Woman: Myths and Legends of the Aztecs* (New York: Quill/Wm. Morrow, 1984), 29–32.

13. "Hale-Bopp Brings Closure to Heaven's Gate," Heaven's Gate, accessed February 22, 2016, http://www .heavensgate.com/misc/intro.htm.

CHAPTER 2
THE DARK SIDE OF THE QUEST

1. Woody Allen, AZQuotes.com, accessed January 20, 2016, http://www.azquotes.com/quote/552998.

2. "The CI Advantage," Cryonics Institute, accessed February 22, 2016, http://www.cryonics.org/the-ci-advantage/.

3. Ibid.

4. Ibid.

5. Ibid.

6. Ibid.

7. Alexander Lazarevich, "The Technology of Immortality," accessed February 22, 2016, http://technocosm.narod .ru/e/wg_e.htm.

8. Ibid.

9. Sebastian Anthony, "What Is Transhumanism, or, What Does It Mean to Be Human?", ExtremeTech, April 1, 2013, accessed February 22, 2016, http://www .extremetech.com/extreme/152240-what-is -transhumanism-or-what-does-it-mean-to-be-human.

10. Michael Snyder, "Transhumanism: An Attempt to Use Technology to Turn Men Into Gods," InfoWars.com, May 5, 2015, accessed February 22, 2016, http://www .infowars.com/transhumanism-an-attempt-to-use -technology-to-turn-men-into-gods/.

11. Ray Kurzweil, "Ray Kurzweil: This Is Your Future," CNN.com, December 26, 2013, accessed February 22, 2016, http://edition.cnn.com/2013/12/10/business /ray-kurzweil-future-of-human-life/index.html.

12. Karl A. Drlica, *Double-Edged Sword: The Promises and Risks of the Genetic Revolution* (Reading, MA: Helix/ Addison-Wesley, 1994), 3.

13. Ibid.

14. Ibid., 84–85.

15. "About Genetic Selection," Genetics and Society, accessed January 18, 2016, http://www.geneticsandsociety.org /section.php?id=82.

16. Albert Einstein, "The Real Problem Is in the Hearts of Men," *New York Times*, June 23, 1946, 44.

17. Elizabeth Landau, "Studies Show 'Dark Chapter' of Medical Research," CNN, October 1, 2010, accessed February 22, 2016, http://www.cnn.com/2010/HEALTH/10/01 /guatemala.syphilis.tuskegee/.

Chapter 3
How Long Can We Live?

1. Steven Goodman, "How Many People Live to 100 Across the Globe?" *The Centenarian*, December 3, 2015, accessed December 22, 2015, http://www.thecentenarian.co.uk /how-many-people-live-to-hundred-across-the-globe.html.

2. "Japan's Centenarian Population Tops 60,000 for First Time," *Japan Times*, September 11, 2015, accessed December 22, 2015, http://www.japantimes.co.jp /news/2015/09/11/national/japans-centenarian -population-tops-60000-first-time/#.VnlzgPkrJph.

3. "Global Health Observatory Data Repository: Life Expectancy," World Health Organization, accessed

December 22, 2015, http://apps.who.int/gho/data/node. main.688?lang=en.

4. Jack Moore, "Two Numbers: Japan Has More Than 60,000 Centenarians, and Tokyo Can't Afford Their Gifts," *Newsweek*, September 23, 2015, accessed January 21, 2016, http://www.newsweek.com/2015/10/02 /turning-100-japan-getting-old-375556.html.

5. Brad Darrach, "The War on Aging," *Life*, October 1992, 36.

6. Moore, "Two Numbers: Japan Has More Than 60,000 Centenarians, and Tokyo Can't Afford Their Gifts."

7. "Global Health Observatory Data Repository: Life Expectancy."

8. Berkeley.edu, "Life Expectancy in the USA, 1900–98, Men and Women," accessed February 22, 2016, http:// demog.berkeley.edu/~andrew/1918/figure2.html.

9. Jennifer M. Ortman, Victoria A Velkoff, and Howard Hogan, "An Aging Nation: The Older Population in the United States," United States Census Bureau, May 2014, accessed January 21, 2016, https://www.census.gov/prod /2014pubs/p25-1140.pdf.

10. J. A. Brody et al., "Epidemiology and Aging: Maximum Reproductive Age Unaffected by Increased Life Expectancy in the Twentieth Century," *Aging Clinical and Experimental Research* 10 (1998): 170–171.

11. The birth rate in the United States is 1.46 percent, roughly 3,950,000 births per year. According to the CDC (www.cdc.gov) in Atlanta there were a total of 972,165 legal abortions in 1999 (346,864 before eight weeks of gestation and 625,301 after eight weeks of gestation).

    New laboratory technology has uncovered a higher rate of miscarriages than earlier thought. The consensus among the experts now is that pregnancies are interrupted naturally between 30 percent and 50 percent of the time (http://www.babycenter.com/0_miscarriage -signs-causes-and-treatment_252.bc). The majority of them happen unbeknownst to women; they appear as "late" menstrual periods, but in fact what happened were micro-abortions (miscarriages), most of them due to congenital anomalies. Once a woman is aware of a pregnancy, the rate of miscarriage drops significantly; 15 to 25 percent of known pregnancies end in miscarriage (http://www.webmd.com/baby/guide/pregnancy-miscarriage). Since only knowing pregnant women request abortions, 75 to 85 percent of the 699,202 aborted children in 2012, between 524,401 and 594,321, should have produced normal children (http://www.cdc.gov/reproductivehealth/data_stats/).

If life expectancy is the average of all deaths in a single year, including accidents, murder, and prenatal deaths (fetal deaths after 30 weeks, because they have an extremely good chance of survival), then, as strict actuary studies demand, abortions should be counted. As you can imagine, in the soup of numbers, 699,202 has a tremendous impact. In addition to raising death rates, abortions raise infant mortality. Infant mortality for 2013 was 5.96 deaths per 1,000 live births, or .596 percent (http://www.cdc.gov/nchs/fastats/deaths.htm). With abortion considered, this raises to a whopping 21.596 percent. This crushes the touted "social gain" claim that life expectancy is now 79 in the United States (with pro-choice laws) (http://apps.who.int/gho/data/view.main.680?lang=en) and supports Carl Sagan's statement that what really improves life expectancy is love for our children.

Even though these numbers might not affect our personal life expectancy, they speak volumes about our social fiber, when we consider that entire cultures, even empires, have been destroyed due to loss of values, especially when it comes to the value of life.

12. "Life Expectancy: Data by Country," World Health Organization, accessed January 19, 2016, http://apps.who.int/gho/data/view.main.680?lang=en.

13. Ibid.

14. D. Harman, "Aging: Phenomena and Theories," *Annals of the New York Academy of Sciences* 854 (November 20, 1998): 1–7.

15. K. Schmidt, "Physiology and Pathophysiology of Senescence," *International Journal for Vitamin and Nutrition Research* 69, no. 3 (1999): 150–153.

16. D. W. E. Smith, "Evolution of Longevity in Mammals," *Mechanisms of Aging and Development* 81 (1995): 51–60.

17. Francisco Contreras, *Health in the 21st Century* (Chula Vista, CA: Interpacific, 1997), 29.

18. M. L. Pardue and P. G. DeBaryshe, "Telomeres and Telomerase: More Than the End of the Line," *Chromosoma* 108 (1999): 73–82.

19. Darrach, "The War on Aging."

20. T. J. Moore, "Genetic Roulette: Figuring the Odds on Your Longevity Inheritance," *MDX Health Digest*.

21. Darrach, "War on Aging," 38.

22. Contreras, *Health in the 21st Century*, 35.

23. Denham Harman, "Aging: A Theory Based on Free Radical and Radiation Chemistry," *Journal of Gerontology II* (1956): 298–300; Denham Harman, "The Aging Process," *Proceedings of the National Academy of Sciences USA* 78 (1981): 7123–7128.

24. R. S. Sohal and R. Weindruch, "Oxidative Stress, Caloric Restriction and Aging," *Science* 273 (1996): 59–63.

25. Free radicals have been implicated in more than a hundred disease conditions in humans, including arthritis, endotoxic and hemorrhagic shock (J. Barroso-Aranda et al., "Neutrophil Activation, Tumor Necrosis Factor, and Survival After Endotoxic and Hemorrhagic Shock," *Journal of Cardiovascular Pharmacology* 25, supp. 2 [1995]: 523–529), atherosclerosis (J. L. Wiztum, "The Oxidation Hypothesis of Atherosclerosis," *Lancet* 344 [1994]: 793–798), ischemia and reperfusion injury of many tissues (G. A. Cordia et al., "Detection of Oxidative DNA Damage to Ischemia Reperfused Rat Hearts by 8-Hydroxydeoxyguanosine Formation," *Molecular Cell Cardiology* 30 [1998]: 1939–1944), Alzheimer's and Parkinson's disease (D. Harman, "Free Radical Theory of Aging: Alzheimer's Disease Pathogenisis," *Age* 18 [1995]: 97–119; C. W. Olanow, "Oxidation Reactions

in Parkinson's Disease," *Neurology* 40, supp. 3 [1990]: 32–37), tumor promotion and carcinogenesis (D. I. Feig et al., "Reactive Oxygen Species in Tumorigenisis," *Cancer Research* 54, supp. [1994]: 1890–1894), and AIDS (B. Halliwell and C. E. Cross, "Reactive Oxygen Species, Antioxidants and Acquired Immunodeficiency Syndrome," *Archives of Internal Medicine* 157 [1991]: 29–32).

26. J. P. Kehner, "Free Radicals as Mediators of Tissue Injury and Disease," *Critical Reviews in Toxicology* 23 (1993): 21–48.

CHAPTER 4
LOSE WEIGHT AND LIVE LONGER

1. Carroll E. Simcox, comp., *4400 Quotations for Christian Communications* (Grand Rapids: Baker, 1991), 111.

2. C. M. McCay, L. A. Maynard, G. Sperling, and L. L. Barnes, "Retarded Growth, Life Span, Ultimate Body Size and Age Changes in the Albino Rat Feeding Diet Restricted Calories," *Journal of Nutrition* 18 (1939): 1–13.

3. Leon Chaitow, "Natural Life Extension: Experimental Evidence of Life Extension," accessed January 21, 2016, http://www.healthy.net/scr/article.aspx?id=1222.

4. Ibid.

5. Gregory M. Fahy, "Aging Revealed!" *Life Extension*, November 1999, accessed January 21, 2016, http://www.lifeextension.com/Magazine/1999/11/cover/Page-01?p=1.

6. Ibid.

7. Ibid.

8. Ibid.

9. Ibid.

10. Chaitow, "Natural Life Extension: Experimental Evidence of Life Extension,"

11. Ibid.

12. Charles Thomas, *Retardation of Aging and Disease by Dietary Restriction* (Springfield, IL: 1998).

13. Zhi-Chien Ho, "A Study of Longevity and Protein Requirements of Individuals 90 to 112 Years Old in

Southern China," *Journal of Applied Nutrition* 34, no. 1 (1982): 12–23.

14. Richard L. Hill, "Research on Aging Looks at Effects of Cutting Calories," *The Oregonian*, January 22, 1999.

15. Roy L. Walford et al., "Calorie Restriction in Biosphere 2: Alterations in Physiologic, Hematologic, Hormonal, and Biochemical Parameters in Humans Restricted for a 2-Year Period," *Journals of Gerontology: Biological Sciences and Medical Sciences* 57, no. 6 (2002): B211–B224.

16. "Researchers Expand Diet and Aging Study," World Health Network, Reuters, July 21, 1999.

17. Ibid.

18. A. Turturro and R. W. Hart, "Caloric Restriction and Its Effects on Molecular Parameters, Especially DNA Repair," in L. Fishbein, ed., *Biological Effects of Dietary Restriction* (New York: Springer-Verlag, 1991), 185–190.

19. T. P. Szatrowski and C. F. Nathan, "Production of Large Amounts of Hydrogen Peroxide by Human Tumor Cells," *Cancer Research* 51 (1991): 794–798.

20. M. G. Simic and D. S. Bergtold, "Urinary Biomarkers of Oxidative DNA Base Damage and Human Caloric Intake," in Fishbein, *Biological Effects of Dietary Restriction*, 217–225.

21. "Low-Cal Diet Blocks Aging Genes," World Health Network, Reuters, August 26, 1999.

22. "Researchers Expand Diet and Aging Study."

23. Ibid.

24. Richard Weindruch, "Influences of Calorie Intake on Aging and Cancer," UW–Madison Institute on Aging.

25. Ibid.

26. Hill, "Research on Aging Looks at Effects of Cutting Calories."

27. Ibid.

28. "Researchers Expand Diet and Aging Study."

29. Hill, "Research on Aging Looks at Effects of Cutting Calories."

CHAPTER 5
EATING FOR LONGEVITY

1. Darrach, "The War on Aging."
2. "Japanese Reaching 100 Hit Record High," World Health Network.
3. W. J. Craig, "Phytochemicals: Guardians of Our Health," *Journal of the American Dietetic Association* 97, supp. 2 (1997): 199S–204S.
4. E. J. Schaefer and M. E. Brosseau, "Diet, Lipoproteins, and Coronary Heart Disease," *Endocrinology and Metabolism Clinics of North America* 27, no. 3 (1998): 711–32.
5. F. B. Hu et al., "Dietary Saturated Fats and Their Food Sources in Relation to the Risk of Coronary Heart Disease in Women," *American Journal of Clinical Nutrition* 70 (1999): 1001–1008.
6. R. P. Mensink and M. B. Katan, "Effect of Dietary Trans Fatty Acids on High-Density and Low-Density Lipoprotein Cholesterol Levels in Healthy Subjects," *New England Journal of Medicine* 323 (1990): 439–445.
7. G. M. Wardlaw and T. J. Snook, "Effect of Diets High in Butter, Corn Oil, or High-Oleic Acid Sunflower Oil or Serum Lipids and Apolipoproteins in Men," *American Journal of Clinical Nutrition* 51 (1990): 815–822; P. Mata et al., "Effect of Dietary Monounsaturated Fatty Acids on Plasma Lipoproteins and Apoliproteins in Women," *American Journal of Clinical Nutrition* 56 (1992): 77–82.
8. Schaefer and Brosseau, "Diet, Lipoproteins, and Coronary Heart Disease."
9. P. J. Nestel, "Fish Oil and Cardiovascular Disease: Lipids and Arterial Function," *American Journal of Clinical Nutrition* 71, supp. (2000): 228S–231S; L. A. Harker et al., "Interruption of Vascular Thrombus Formation and Vascular Lesion Formation by Dietary N=3 Fatty Acids in Fish Oil in Non-Human Primates," *Circulation* 87 (1993): 1017–1029.
10. J. Slavin, D. Jacobs, and L. Marquant, "Whole-Grain Consumption and Chronic Disease: Protective Mechanism," *Nutrition and Cancer* 27 (1997): 14–21.

11. B. N. Ames, "Micronutrients Prevent Cancer and Delay Aging," *Toxicology Letters* 102–103 (December 28, 1998): 5–18.

12. J. A. Joseph et al., "Reversals of Age-Related Declines in Neuronal Signal Transduction, Cognitive, and Motor Behavioral Deficits With Blueberry, Spinach or Strawberry Dietary Supplementation," *Journal of Neuroscience* 19, no. 18 (1999): 8114–8121.

13. Walter J. Crinnon, "Are Organic Foods Really Healthier for You?", *Organic Gardening Almanac* (Woodbury, MN: Llewelyn, 1995).

14. Ibid.

15. Ibid.

16. Ibid.

17. Ibid. Also, "Organic Produce: New Consumer Reports Study Finds: It Really Is Different," *Consumer News*, December 15, 1997.

18. S. Franceschi et al., "Tomatoes and the Risk of Digestive-Tract Cancers," *International Journal of Cancer* 59 (1994): 181–184.

19. B. Haber, "The Mediterranean Diet: A View From History," *American Journal of Clinical Nutrition* 66, supp. (1997):1053S–1057S.

20. A. Trichopoulou and P. Lagiou, "Healthy Traditional Mediterranean Diet: An Expression of Culture, History and Lifestyle," *Nutrition Reviews* 55, no. 11 (1997): 383–389.

21. M. Gronbaek et al., "Mortality Associated With Moderate Intakes of Wine, Beer, or Spirits," *British Medical Journal* 310 (1995): 1165–1169.

22. G. J. Soleas, E. P. Diamandis, and D. M. Goldberg, "Wine as a Biological Fluid: History, Production, and Role in Disease Prevention," *Journal of Clinical Laboratory Analysis* 11 (1997): 287–313.

23. Gronbaek et al., "Mortality Associated with Moderate Intakes of Wine, Beer, or Spirits."

24. S. V. Nigdikar et al., "Consumption of Red Wine Polyphenols Reduces the Susceptibility of Low-Density

Lipoprotein to Oxidation in Vivo," *American Journal of Clinical Nutrition* 68 (1998): 258–265; M. Sarafini et al., "Alcohol-Free Red Wine Enhances Plasma Antioxidant Capacity in Humans," *Journal of Nutrition* 128 (1998): 1003–1007; A. Lavy et al., "Effect of Dietary Supplementation of Red Wine on Human Blood Chemistry, Hematology and Coagulation: Favorable Effect of Red Wine on Plasma-High Density Lipoprotein," *Annals of Nutrition and Metabolism* 38 (1994): 287–294.

25. Soleas, Diamandis, and Goldberg, "Wine as a Biological Fluid: History Production, and Role in Disease Prevention."

26. Ibid.

27. J. Constant, "Alcohol, Ischemic Heart Disease, and the French Paradox," *Clinical Cardiology* 20 (1997): 420–424.

28. H. Mukhtar and N. Ahmad, "Mechanism of Cancer Chemopreventive Activity of Green Tea," *Proceedings of the Society for Experimental Biology and Medicine* 220, no. 4 (1999): 234–238.

29. T. O. Cheng, "Antioxidants in Chinese Green Tea," *Journal of the American College of Cardiology* 31, no. 5 (1998): 1214.

30. S. Uchida et al., "Effects of Epigallocatechin—3-O-Gallete (Green Tea Tannin) on Life Span of Stroke-Prone Spontaneously Hypertensive Rats," *Clinical and Experimental Pharmacology and Physiology* 22, supp. 1 (1995): 302S–303S.

31. G. E. Fraser, "Nut Consumption, Lipids, and Risk of a Coronary Event," *Clinical Cardiology* 22, supp. 3 (1999): 11–15; P. M. Kris-Etherton et al., "Nuts and Their Bioactive Constituents: Effects on Serum Lipids and Other Factors That Affect Disease Risk," *American Journal of Clinical Nutrition* 70, supp. (1999): 504S–511S.

32. G. E. Fraser et al., "A Possible Protective Effect of Nut Consumption on Risk of Coronary Heart Disease," *Archives of Internal Medicine* 152 (1992): 1416–1424; L. Brown et al., "Nut Consumption and Risk of Recurrent

Coronary Heart Disease (Abstract)," *FASEB Journal* 13, no. 4–5 (1999): A538.

33. Ibid.

34. G. E. Fraser, K. D. Lindsted, and W. L. Beeson, "Effect of Risk Factor Values on Lifetime Risk of an Age at First Coronary Event," *American Journal of Epidemiology* 142 (1995): 746–758.

35. A. L. Waterhouse, J. R. Shirley, and J. L. Donovan, "Antioxidants in Chocolate," *Lancet* 348 (1996): 834.

36. K. Kondo et al., "Inhibition of LDL Oxidation by Cocoa," *Lancet* 348 (1996): 154.

37. T. P. A. Devasagayam et al., "Caffeine as an Antioxidant: Inhibition of Lipid Peroxidation Induced by Reactive Oxygen Species," *Biochimica et Biophysica Acta* 1282 (1996): 63–70.

38. J. H. Weisburger et al., "Inhibition of PhIP, Mutagenicity by Caffeine, Lycopene, Daidzein and Ginseng," *Mutation Research* 416 (1998): 125–128.

39. Qing Yang, "Gain Weight by 'Going Diet?' Artificial Sweeteners and the Neurobiology of Sugar Cravings," *Yale Journal of Biology and Medicine* 83, no. 2 (June 2010): 101–108.

40. Julian Whitaker, *Health and Healing* 7, no. 11 (November 1977).

Chapter 6
Extend Your Life With Vitamins

1. The annual per capita consumption of refined sugar in the United States will have increased from 0 in the middle of the eighteenth century to about 100 pounds by the end of the twentieth century. Fat consumption has increased dramatically from about 20 percent of the energy intake in the middle of the nineteenth century to about 50 percent today, despite the fact that people today need much less energy because of generally reduced levels of physical activity. S. Bengmark, "Ecoimmunonutrition: A Challenge for the Third Millennium," *Nutrition* 14, no. 7–8 (1998): 563–572.

2. *Encyclopaedia Britannica*, s.v. "Beriberi," accessed January 19, 2016, http://www.britannica.com/science/beriberi.

3. Ibid.; also, *The Columbia Encyclopedia*, 6th ed. (2000), s.v. "Funk, Casimir"; Funk, Casimir, www.bartleby.com/65/fy /Funk-Cas.

4. Jean Carper, *Stop Aging Now!* (New York: HarperCollins, 1996), 49.

5. Ibid., 50.

6. Ibid.

7. B. Frei, L. England, and B. N. Ames, "Ascorbate Is an Outstanding Antioxidant in Human Blood Plasma," *Proceedings of the National Academy of Sciences* 86 (1989): 6377–6381.

8. D. Harats et al., "Effect of Vitamin C and E Supplementation of Susceptibility of Plasma Lipoproteins to Preoccupation Induced by Acute Smoking," *Atherosclerosis* 85 (1990): 47–54.

9. H. B. Stahelin, "The Impact of Antioxidants on Chronic Disease in Aging and in Old Age," *International Journal for Vitamin and Nutrition Research* 69, no. 3 (1999): 146–149.

10. Carper, *Stop Aging Now!*, 57.

11. V. G. Bezlepkin, N. P. Sirota, and A. L Gaziev, "The Prolongation of Survival in Mice by Dietary Antioxidants Depends on Their Age by the Start of Feeding This Diet," *Mechanisms of Aging and Development* 92, no. 2–3 (1996): 227–234.

12. M. Corwin et al., "Studies of the Mode of Action of Vitamin E in Stimulating T-Cell Mitogenesis," *Scandinavian Journal of Immunology* 14 (1981): 565–571.

13. E. B. Rimm et al., "Vitamin E Consumption and the Risk of Coronary Heart Disease in Men," *New England Journal of Medicine* 328 (1993): 1450–1456.

14. S. E. Edmons et al., "Putative Analgesic Activity of Repeated Oral Doses of Vitamin E in the Treatment of Rheumatoid Arthritis: Results of a Prospective Placebo-Controlled, Double Blind Trial," *Annals of Rheumatoid Disease* 56 (1997): 649–655.

15. S. G. Post, "Future Scenarios for the Prevention and Delay of Alzheimer Disease Onset in High-Risk Groups. An Ethical Perspective," *American Journal of Preventative Medicine* 16, no. 2 (1999): 105–110.

16. I. Jialal et al., "The Effect of Alpha-Tocopherol Supplementation on LDL Oxidation: A Dose-Response Study," *Arteriosclerosis, Thrombosis, and Vascular Biology* 15 (1995): 190–198.

17. Ibid.

18. B. P. Yu et al., "Can Antioxidant Supplementation Slow the Aging Process?", *Biofactors* 7, no. 1–2 (1998): 93–101.

19. Carper, *Stop Aging Now!*, 59.

20. J. W. Jama et al., "Dietary Antioxidants and Cognitive Function in a Population-Based Sample of Older Persons. The Rotterdam Study," *American Journal of Epidemiology* 144 (1996): 275–280.

21. Carper, *Stop Aging Now!*, 66.

22. Ibid.

23. Ibid.

24. Ibid., 70.

25. Ibid., 77.

26. Chasan-Taber et al., "A Prospective Study of Folate and Vitamin B_6 and Risk of Myocardial Infarction in US Physicians," *Journal of the American College of Nutrition* 15 (1996): 136–143; E. B. Rimm et al., "Folate and Vitamin B_6 from Diet and Supplements in Relation to Risk of Coronary Heart Disease Among Women," *Journal of the American Medical Association* 279, no. 5 (1998): 359–364.

27. Naurath et al., "Effects of Vitamin B_{12}, Folate and Vitamin B_6 Supplements in Elderly People with Normal Serum Vitamin Concentrations," *Lancet* 346 (1995): 85–89; K. L. Tucker et al., "Dietary Intake Pattern Relates to Plasma Folate and Homocysteine Concentrations in the Framingham Heart Study," *Journal of Nutrition* 126, no. 2 (1996): 3025–3031.

28. C. J. Boushey et al., "A Quantitative Assessment of Plasma Homocysteine as a Risk Factor for Vascular Disease: Probable Benefits of Increasing Folic Acid Intakes,"

Journal of the American Medical Association 274 (1995): 1049–1057; O. Nygard et al., "Plasma Homocysteine Levels and Mortality in Patients With Coronary Artery Disease," *New England Journal of Medicine* 337 (1997): 230–236.

29. Carper, *Stop Aging Now!*, 78.

CHAPTER 7
MINING MINERALS FOR LONGEVITY

1. "What Americans Eat—for Better, for Worse," United States Department of Agriculture, April 1995, accessed January 21, 2016, http://www.ars.usda.gov/is/np/fnrb/fnrb495.htm#eat.
2. G. W. Evans and L. Meyer, "Chromium Picolinate Increases Longevity," *AGE* 15 (1992): 134.
3. Carper, *Stop Aging Now!*, 81.
4. Ibid.
5. D. L. Hasten et al., "Dosage Effects on Chromium Picolinate on Body Composition," *FASEB Journal* 8 (1994): A194; R. I. Press, J. Geller, and G. W. Evans, "The Effect of Chromium Picolinate on Serum Cholesterol and Apolipoprotein Fractions in Human Subjects," *Western Journal of Medicine* 152 (1990): 41–45.
6. Carper, *Stop Aging Now!*, 83.
7. Ibid.
8. H. D. Foster and L. Zhang, "Longevity and Selenium Deficiency: Evidence From the People's Republic of China," *Science of the Total Environment* 170, no. 1–2 (1995): 133–139.
9. L. C. Clark et al., "Effects of Selenium Supplementation for Cancer Prevention in Patients With Carcinoma of the Skin: A Randomized Controlled Trial," *Journal of the American Medical Association* 276 (1996): 1957–1963.
10. Carper, *Stop Aging Now!*, 117.
11. Ibid., 118.
12. C. Fortes, "Aging, Zinc and Cell-Mediated Immune Response," *Aging Clinical and Experimental Research* 7 (1995): 75–76.

13. Carper, *Stop Aging Now!*, 92.

14. R. L. Walford, *The Immunological Theory of Aging* (Copenhagen: Munksgaard, 1969), 1–248.

15. A. Sbarbati et al., "Effect of Dietary Supplementation With Zinc Sulfate on the Aging Process: A Study Using High Field Intensity MRI and Chemical Shift Imaging," *Biomedicine and Pharmacotherapy* 52, no. 10 (1998): 454–458.

16. Carper, *Stop Aging Now!*, 95–96.

17. Ibid., 97.

18. Maureen Kennedy Salaman, *All Your Health Questions Answered Naturally* (n.p.: Maximum Living Inc., 1998), 119.

19. Carper, *Stop Aging Now!*, 139.

20. J. R. Huertas et al., "Virgin Olive Oil and Coenzyme Q_{10} Protect Heart Mitochondria From Peroxidative Damage During Aging," *Biofactor* 9, no. 2–4 (1999): 337–343.

21. R. Aejmaelaeus et al., "Ubiquinol-10 and Total Peroxy Radical Trapping Capacity of LDL Lipopropteins During Aging and the Effects of Q_{10} Supplementation," *Molecular Aspects of Medicine* 18, supp. (1997): 113S–120S.

22. A. Kontush et al., "Plasma Ubiquinol-10 Is Decreased in Patients With Hyperlipidaemia," *Atherosclerosis* 129 (1997): 119–126; S. T. Sinatra, "Care, Cancer and Coenzyme Q_{10}," *Journal of American College of Cardiology* 33, no. 3 (1999): 897–898.

23. T. Blatt et al, "Modulation of Oxidative Stresses in Human Aging Skin," *Zeitschrift fur Gerontologie und Geriatrie* 32, no. 2 (1999): 83–88.

24. R. K. Chopra et al., "Relative Bioavailability of Coenzyme Q_{10} Formulations in Human Subjects," *International Journal for Vitamin and Nutrition Research* 68 (1998): 109–113.

25. D. Kromhout et al., "The Inverse Relation between Fish Consumption and 20-Year Mortality From Coronary Heart Disease," *New England Journal of Medicine* 312 (1985): 1205–1209.

26. L. A. Horrocks and Y. K. Yeo, "Health Benefits of Docosahexaenoic Acid (DHA)," *Pharmacological Research* 40, no. 3 (1999): 211–225.

27. Ibid.

28. F. N. Hepburn et al., "Provisional Tablets on the Content of Omega-3 Fatty Acids and Other Fat Components of Selected Foods," *Journal of the American Diet Association* 86 (1986): 788–793.

29. P. M. Kris-Etherton et al., "Polyunsaturated Fatty Acids in the Food Chain in the United States," *American Journal of Clinical Nutrition* 71, supp. (2000): 179S–188S.

30. Ibid.

31. Ibid.

32. C. Von Schacky, "N-3 Fatty Acids and the Prevention of Coronary Atherosclerosis," *American Journal of Clinical Nutrition* 71, supp. (2000): 224S–227S.

33. J. X. Kang and A. Leaf, "Prevention of Fatal Arrhythmias by Poly-Unsaturated Fatty Acids," *American Journal of Clinical Nutrition* 71, supp. (2000): 202S–207S.

34. W. E. Connor, "Importance of N-3 Fatty Acids in Health and Disease," *American Journal of Clinical Nutrition* 71, supp. (2000): 171S–175S.

35. F. Driss et al., "Inhibition of Platelet Aggregation and Tromboxane Synthesis After Intake of Small Amount of Eicosapentaenoic Acid," *Thrombosis Research* 36 (1984): 389–396.

36. C. M. Albert et al., "Fish Consumption and Risk of Sudden Cardiac Death," *Journal of the American Medical Association* 279 (1998): 23–27.

37. S. L. Connor and W. E. Connor, "Are Fish Oils Beneficial in the Prevention and Treatment of Coronary Artery Disease?" *American Journal of Clinical Nutrition* 66, supp. (1997): 1020S–1031S.

38. T. Moriguchi, H. Saito, and N. Nishiyama, "Aged Garlic Extract Prolongs Longevity and Improves Spatial Memory Deficit in Senescence-Accelerated Mouse," *Biological and Pharmaceutical Bulletin* 19, no. 2 (1996): 305–307.

39. Carper, *Stop Aging Now!*, 163.
40. N. Ide and B. H. S. Lau, "Garlic Compounds Protect Vascular Endothelial Cells From Oxidized Low-Density Lipoprotein-Induced Injury," *Journal of Pharmacology* 49 (1997): 908–911.
41. L. D. Lawson et al., "Inhibition of Whole Blood Platelet Aggregation by Compounds in Garlic Clove Extracts and Commercial Garlic Products," *Thrombosis Research* 65 (1992): 141–156.
42. E. M. Schaffer et al., "Garlic and Associated Allyl Sulfur Components Inhibit N-Methyl-N-Nitrosourea-Induced Rat Mammary Carcinogenesis," *Cancer Letters* 102 (1996): 199–204.
43. K. Prasad et al., "Antioxidant Activity of Allicin, and Active Principle in Garlic," *Molecular and Cellular Biochemistry* 148 (1995): 183–189.
44. R. S. Feldberg et al., "In Vitro Mechanism of Inhibition of Bacterial Cell Growth by Allicin," *Antimicrobial Agents Chemotherapy* 32 (1988): 1763–1768.
45. R. A. Nagourney, "Garlic: Medicinal Food or Nutritious Medicine?" *Journal of Medicinal Food* 1, no. 1 (1998): 13–28.
46. J. C. Winter, "The Effects of an Extract of Ginkgo Biloba, Egb761, on Cognitive Behavior and Longevity in the Rat," *Physiology and Behavior* 63, no. 3 (1998): 425–433.
47. F. G. De Feudis, *Ginkgo Biloba Extract (Egb 761): Pharmacological Activities and Clinical Applications*, F. C. De Feudis, ed. (Paris: Editions Scientifiques Elservier, 1991), 7–146.
48. G. S. Rai, C. Shovlin, and K. A. Wesnes, "A Double-Blind, Placebo-Controlled Study of Ginkgo Biloba Extract ('Tanakan') in Elderly Outpatients With Mild to Moderate Memory Impairment," *Current Medical Research and Opinion* 12, no. 6 (1991): 350–355.
49. R. Sikora et al., "Ginkgo Biloba Extract in the Therapy of Erectile Dysfunction," *Journal of Urology* 141, Abstract (1989): 188A; A. J. Cohen et al., "Ginkgo Biloba for

Antidepressant-Induced Sexual Dysfunction," *Journal of Sex and Marital Therapy* 24, no. 2 (1998): 139–143.

50. J. G. Shen and D. Y. Zhou, "Efficiency of Ginkgo Biloba Extract (EGb761) in Antioxidant Protection Against Myocardial Ischemia and Reperfusion Injury," *Biochemistry and Molecular Biology International* 35, no. 1 (1995): 125–134; S. Piertri et al., "Cardioprotective and Antioxidant Effects of the Terpenoid Constituents of Ginkgo Biloba Extract (Egb 761)," *Journal of Molecular and Cellular Cardiology* 29 (1997): 733–742.

51. D. Zhang et al., "Ginseng Extract Scavenges Hydroxyl Radical and Protects Unsaturated Fatty Acids From Decomposition Caused by Iron—Mediated Lipid Peroxidation," *Free Radical Biology and Medicine* 20, no. 1 (1996): 145–150.

52. U. Banarjee and J. A. Izquierdo, "Antistress and Anti-Fatigue Properites of Panax Ginseng: Comparison With Piracetam," *Acta Physiologica Latino Americana* 32, no. 4 (1982): 277–285.

53. B. H. Lee et al., "In Vitro Antigenotoxic Activity of Novel Ginseng Saponin Metabolites Formed by Intestinal Bacteria," *Planta Medica* 64, no. 6 (1998): 500–503.

54. H. Sorensen and J. Sonne, "A Double-Masked Study of the Effects of Ginseng on Cognitive Functions," *Current Therapeutic Research—Clinical and Experimental* 57, no. 12 (1996): 959–968.

55. X. Chen and T. J. F. Lee, "Gensenosides-Induced Nitric Oxide Mediated Relaxation of the Rabbit Corpus Cavernosum," *British Journal of Pharmacology* 115 (1995): 573–580; C. N. Gillis, "Panax Ginseng Pharmacology: A Nitric Oxide Link?", *Biochemical Pharmacology* 54 (1997): 1–8.

56. M. Sato et al., "Cardioprotective Effects of Grape Seed Proanthocyanidin Against Ischemic Reperfusion Injury," *Journal of Molecular and Cellular Cardiology* 31 (1999): 1289–1297.

57. C. Corbe, J. P. Boissin and A. Siou, "Light Vision and Chorioretinal Circulation. Study of the Effect of

Procyanidolic Oligomers," *J. Fr. Ophthalmol.* 11 (1988): 453–460; S. D. Ray et al., "A Novel Proanthocyanidin IH 636 Grape Seed Extract Increases in Vivo Bcl-XL Expression and Prevents Acetaminophen-Induced Programmed and Unprogrammed Cell Death in Mouse Liver," *Archives of Biochemistry and Biophysics* 369, no. 1 (1999): 42–58.

CHAPTER 8
DISCOVERING ENZYMES AND HORMONES

1. "Cellular Fountain of Youth Works, Scientists Conclude," January 13, 1998, accessed 2000, www.mercurycenter .com/scitech.center/agingo1498.
2. Ibid.
3. Ibid.
4. Ibid.
5. J. Travis, "Missing Enzyme Incites Cancer Debate," *ScienceNews* 152, no. 15 (October 1997), 228.
6. A. Giustina et al., "Growth Hormone Treatment in Aging: State of the Art and Perspectives," *Aging Clinical and Experimental Research* 9, supp. to no. 4. (1997): 73; E. Corpas, S. M. Harman, and M. R. Blackman, "Growth Hormone and Human Aging," *Endocrine Reviews* 14 (1993): 20–30.
7. Ibid.
8. Douglas Skrecky, "More Information About Growth Hormone: The Cause of Aging," North Dakota State University Experiment, accessed January 21, 2016, www .vespro.com/health/moreinfo/dakota.html.
9. D. Rudman et al., "Effect on Human Growth Hormone in Men Over 60 Years Old," *New England Journal of Medicine* 323 (1990): 1–6.
10. "Human Growth Hormone—Is It the Fountain of Youth?" VesPro Life Sciences, accessed January 21, 2016, www.vespro.com/health/human.html.
11. "Measuring Growth Hormone in the Body," VesPro Life Sciences, accessed January 21, 2016, http://hgh.vespro .com/measuring.html.
12. Ibid.

13. Gabe Mirkin, "Growth Hormone and Longevity," accessed January 19, 2016, http://www.drmirkin.com /archive/6947.html.
14. R. J. Reiter, "The Aging Pineal Gland and Its Physiological Consequences," *Bioessays* 14 (1992): 169–175.
15. R. J. Reiter et al., "Reactive Oxygen Intermediates, Molecular Damage, and Aging. Relation to Melatonin," *Annals of the New York Academy of Sciences* 854 (1998): 410– 424; T. Uz et al., "Protective Effect of Melatonin Against Hippocampal DNA Damage Induced by Intraperitoneal Administration of Kainate to Rats," *Neuroscience* 73 (1996): 631–636.
16. Reiter et al., "Reactive Oxygen Intermediates, Molecular Damage, and Aging. Relation to Melatonin."
17. K. A. Stokkan et al., "Food Restriction Retards Aging of the Pineal Gland," *Brain Research* 545 (1991): 66–72.
18. W. Pierpaoli and W. Regelson, "Pineal Control of Aging: Effect of Melatonin and Pineal Grafting on Aging Mice," *Proceedings of the National Academy of Sciences USA* 91 (1994): 787–791.
19. Ibid.
20. W. Pierpaoli et al., "The Pineal Control of Aging: The Effects of Melatonin and Pineal Grafting on the Survival of Older Mice," *Annals of the New York Academy of Sciences* 621 (1991): 291–313.
21. Ibid.
22. "Why the Excitement Over Melatonin?", All-Natural, accessed January 21, 2016, www.all-natural.com/melaton .html.
23. D. Dawson and N. Encel, "Melatonin and Sleep in Humans," *Journal of Pineal Research* 15 (1993): 1–12.
24. "Why the Excitement Over Melatonin?"
25. Ibid.
26. D. X. Tan et al., "Both Physiological and Pharmacological Levels of Melatonin Reduce DNA Adduct Formation Induced by the Carcinogen Safrole," *Carcinogenesis* 15 (1994): 615–618.

27. P. Burgger et al., "Impaired Nocturnal Secretion of Melatonin in Coronary Heart Disease," *Lancet* 345 (1995):
1408; T. Y. Chan and P. L. Tang, "Effect of Melatonin
on the Maintenance of Cholesterol Homeostasis in Rats,"
Endocrinology Research 21, no. 3 (1995): 681–696.

28. M. A. Pappolla et al., "Melatonin Prevents Death of Neu-
roblastoma Cells Exposed to Alzheimer Amyloid Pro-
tein," *Journal of Neuroscience* 17 (1997): 1683–1690; J. W.
Miller et al., "Oxidative Damage Caused by Free Radi-
cals Produced During Catecholamine Autoxidation: Pro-
tective Effects of O-Methylation and Melatonin," *Free
Radical Biology and Medicine* 21 (1996): 241–249; D. A.
Acuna-Castroviejo et al., "Melatonin Is Protective Against
MPTP-Induced Striatal and Hippocampal Lesions," *Life
Sciences* 60 (1996): PL23–PL29.

29. J. S. Tenover, "Effects of Testosterone Supplementation
in the Aging Male," *Journal of Clinical Endocrinology and
Metabolism* 75 (1992): 1092–1098; R. J. Urbane et al.,
"Testosterone Administration to Elderly Men Increases
Skeletal Muscle Strength and Protein Synthesis," *Amer-
ican Journal of Physiology* 269 (1995): E820–E826.

30. Ibid.

31. J. L. Tenover, "Testosterone and the Aging Male," *Journal
of Andrology* 18, no. 2 (1997): 103–106.

32. John R. Lee and Virginia Hopkins, *What Your Doctor
May Not Tell You About Menopause* (New York: Warner,
1976).

33. Francisco Contreras, *Women: Your Body and Natural Progesterone* (Chula Vista, CA: Interpacific).

34. "Hormones That Enhance the Effects of Growth Hormone," VesPro Life Sciences, accessed January 21, 2016,
www.vespro.com/health/hormones.html.

35. "In Search of the Fountain of Youth," accessed 2000, www
.angelfire.com/oh2/fountainofyouth.

36. A. J. Morales et al., "Effects of Replacement Dose
of Dehydroepian-Drosterone in Men and Women of
Advancing Age," *Journal of Clinical Endocrinology and
Metabolism* 78 (1994): 1360–1367.

37. A. J. Morales et al., "The Effect of Six Months Treatment With 100 Mg. Daily Dose of Dehydroepiandrosterone (DHEA) or Circulating Sex Steriods, Body Composition and Muscle Strength in Age-Advanced Men and Women," *Clinical Endocrinology* 49 (1998): 421–432.

38. Gregory M. Fahy, "DHEA Extends Lifespan New Analog Ready for Clinical Trials," *Life Extension Magazine*, May 1996, accessed February 23, 2016, http://www .lifeextension.com/magazine/1996/5/event/page-01.

39. Ibid.

CHAPTER 9
EXERCISE: GET MOVING TOWARD LONGEVITY!

1. "Jack Nicklaus Quotes," BrainyQuote.com, accessed January 20, 2016, http://www.brainyquote.com/quotes /authors/j/jack_nicklaus_2.html.

2. P. Thomas, Harvard Health Letter, April 22, 1997, no. 6, 1–3.

3. Ibid.

4. A. La Voie, "Vigorous Exercise Lowers Risk Factors More Than Moderate Activity," *Medical Tribune* 38, no. 4, Family Physician ed. (February 20, 1997): 5.

5. J. E. Brody, "Study Says Exercise Must Be Strenuous to Stretch Lifetime," *New York Times*, April 19, 1995, accessed January 21, 2016, http://www.nytimes.com /1995/04/19/us/study-says-exercise-must-be-strenuous-to -stretch-lifetime.html.

6. "The John Hopkins Prescription for Longevity: Health After 50," *Johns Hopkins Medical Letter* 10 (December 10, 1998): 4–6.

7. *Harvard Men's Health Watch* 12 (July 2 1998): 3–4; Walking to Health.

8. Ibid.

9. "Jogging Might Build Up Your Brain," accessed 2000, www.msnbc.com/news/243509.asp?cp1=1.

10. "Exercise Prescription for Health and Longevity," World Health Network, accessed 2000, www.worldhealth.net /news/exercise3.

11. Ibid.
12. "Jogging Might Build Up Your Brain."
13. Ibid.
14. Jacqueline Stenson, "The Doctor Is In, Moderate Exercise Slashes Stroke Risk," October 8, accessed 2000, www /msnbc.com/news/203390.asp.
15. Ibid.
16. Ibid.
17. Weighty Issues for Seniors, AFAR, accessed 2000, www .afar.org/weight.
18. World Health Network, accessed 2000, www .worldhealth.net/news/exercise3.

Chapter 10
Lifestyle and Longevity:
Overcoming Habits That Steal Years

1. "Dylan Thomas: Quotes," GoodReads, accessed January 20, 2016, http://www.goodreads.com/quotes/93707-i-ve -had-eighteen-straight-whiskies-i-think-that-s-the-record.
2. Jane E. Brody, "7 Deadly Sins of Living Linked to Illness as Well as Mortality," *New York Times*, May 12, 1993, accessed January 21, 2016, http://www.nytimes.com /1993/05/12/health/7-deadly-sins-of-living-linked-to -illness-as-well-as-mortality.html?pagewanted=all.
3. Ibid.
4. Ibid.
5. Honor Whiteman, "Health and Fitness Habits 'Influence Health Over Next Two Decades,'" *Medical News Today*, February 16, 2014, accessed January 21, 2016, http://www .medicalnewstoday.com/articles/272702.php.
6. J. Blyskal, "Longevity: Healthy and Wealthy or Healthy and Wise?" 1993, accessed 2000, www.thrive.net/health /Library?CAD/abstract9662.
7. "For Men Only," Nutrition Action, June 22, 1995, thrive@ health; (5): 1, 4–7; accessed 2000, www.thrive.net/health /Library/CAD/abstract4181.
8. Ibid.

9. Jimmy Carter, *The Virtues of Aging* (New York: Ballantine, 1998), 57.

10. Ibid., 58.

11. Ibid.

12. Ibid.

13. "Banish Bad Health Habits for Good," accessed 2000, www.msnbc.com/news/185857.asp.

14. Ibid.

15. Ibid.

16. Zig Ziglar, *Over the Top* (Nashville: Thomas Nelson, 1997), 93.

17. Ibid., 92.

18. Ibid.

CHAPTER 11
SETTING YOUR ATTITUDE FOR LONGEVITY

1. "Age Quotes," BrainyQuote, accessed January 22, 2016, http://www.brainyquote.com/quotes/quotes/g/georgeburn103932.html?src=t_age.

2. "Attitudes: Key to Health, Happiness & Longevity," accessed February 24, 2016, www.attitudefactor.com.

3. Ibid.

4. Ibid.

5. Ziglar, *Over the Top*, 285.

6. Ibid., 285–86.

7. Ibid., 199.

8. Ibid.

9. Ibid., 200.

10. Yale News, "Thinking Positively About Aging Extends Life More Than Exercise and Not Smoking," July 29, 2002, accessed February 24, 2016, http://news.yale.edu/2002/07/29/thinking-positively-about-aging-extends-life-more-exercise-and-not-smoking.

11. Bernie S. Siegel, *Love, Medicine and Miracles* (New York: Harper & Row, 1986), 35.

12. "William James Quotes," GoodReads.com, accessed January 20, 2016, http://www.goodreads.com

/quotes/374489-the-greatest-revolution-of-our-generation-is
-the-discovery-that.

13. Siegel, *Love, Medicine and Miracles*, 88.

14. Ibid., 81–82.

15. A. Berger, "A Fountain of Youth in Music Class," *New York Times*, June 15, 1999, F8.

16. Siegel, *Love, Medicine and Miracles*, 161.

17. Ibid., 160.

Chapter 12
Laughter and Longevity

1. Christine Overall, *Aging, Death, and Human Longevity: A Philosophical Inquiry* (Los Angeles: University of California Press, 2003), 233.

2. Siegel, *Love, Medicine and Miracles*, 145.

3. Tracy Pipp, "Can Laughter Really Be the Best Medicine?", *Detroit News*, September 30, 1996, accessed 2000, www .detroitnews.com/1996/menu/stories/671318; ScienceDaily.com, "Laughter Remains Good Medicine," April 17, 2009, accessed February 24, 2016, https://www .sciencedaily.com/releases/2009/04/090417084115.htm.

4. Karen S. Peterson, "A Chuckle a Day Does Indeed Help Keep Ills at Bay," *USA Today*, October 31, 1996, 10D.

5. Barry Bittman, "Laughter: A Prescription for Wellness," accessed 2000, www.mind-body.org/laugh.

6. Peterson, "A Chuckle a Day Does Indeed Help Keep Ills at Bay."

7. Ibid.

8. Ibid.

9. Gael Crystal and Patrick Flanagan, "Laughter—Still the Best Medicine," accessed February 24, 2016, http://www .angelfire.com/blues2/pamelyntan703/ARTICLE /article%20pnye%20front/Laughter%20is%20the%20 best%20medicine.htm.

10. Melissa Harlow, "Laughter Heals Body, Stops Stress," *Lariat*, February 12, 1997, accessed February 24, 2016, http://www.baylor.edu/lariatarchives/news .php?action=story&story=10350.

11. Lee Berk and Stanley Tan, "The Laughter-Immune Connection," accessed January 20, 2016, http://www.hospitalclown.com/archives/vol-02/vol-2-1and2/vol2-2berk.PDF.

12. Flanagan, "Laughter—Still the Best Medicine."

13. Berk and Tan, "The Laughter-Immune Connection."

14. Peter Doskoch, "Happily Ever Laughter," PsychologyToday.com, July 1, 1996, accessed February 24, 2016, https://www.psychologytoday.com/articles/199607/happily-ever-laughter.

15. Harlow, "Laughter Heals Body, Stops Stress."

16. Bittman, "Laughter: A Prescription for Wellness."

17. Ibid.

18. Ibid.

19. Ibid.

20. Flanagan, "Laughter—Still the Best Medicine."

21. "Top Ten Causes of Stress—Money—Workplace—Crime," HealthWorks!, accessed 2000, www.allstressedup.com/tacts.

22. Ibid.

23. Patty Wooten, "Humor an Antidote for Stress," *Holistic Nursing Practice* 10, no. 2 (1996): 49–55, accessed January 21, 2016, http://pattywooten.com/images/HumorStressAntidote.pdf.

24. Ibid.

25. Ibid.

26. Ibid.

27. Ibid.

28. Ibid.

29. Ibid.

30. Ibid.

31. G. Williams III, "Longevity: Fatal Emotions," October 1993, accessed 2000, www.thrive.net/health.Library/CAD/abstract8748.

32. "Anger Management: What Is Anger?," accessed 2000, http://home.jxdcb.net.cn/~mccloud/anger.

33. Ibid.

34. "Anger Management: Understanding the Goals of Nega-
    tive Behavior," accessed 2000, http://home.jxdcb.net
    .cn/~mccloud/negative.
35. "Anger Resolution vs. Anger Control," accessed 2000,
    www.teleport.com/~rnbowlkr/anger/resolvscontrol.
36. HealthWorks!, "What Do Your Adrenals and Stress
    Have in Common?", accessed 2000, www.allstressedup
    .com.
37. Ibid.
38. Flanagan, "Laughter—Still the Best Medicine."
39. "Humorous Tombstone Inscriptions," Clemsford History,
    accessed January 21, 2016, http://www.chelmsfordhistory
    .org/humor-cemetery.html

CHAPTER 13
ALL YOU NEED IS LOVE

1. Contreras, *Health in the 21st Century*, 328.
2. Daniel Goleman, "Stress and Isolation Tied to a Reduced
   Life Span," *New York Times*, December 7, 1993, accessed
   January 21, 2016, http://www.nytimes.com/1993/12/07
   /science/stress-and-isolation-tied-to-a-reduced-life-span
   .html.
3. Ibid.
4. Ibid.
5. Siegel, *Love, Medicine and Miracles*, 183.
6. Leo Buscaglia, PhD, has written several books on loving
   relationships, including *Born for Love: Reflections on
   Loving* and *Living, Loving and Learning*.
7. Contreras, *Health in the 21st Century*, 326.
8. Marilyn Elias, "Love Your Parents—Save Their Lives,"
   USA Today, November 18, 1999.
9. Ibid.
10. Siegel, *Love, Medicine and Miracles*, 182–183.
11. Ibid., 199.
12. Ziglar, *Over the Top*, 262.
13. Ibid.
14. Ibid.

15. Ibid.
16. Ibid.

CHAPTER 14
SUCCESSFUL AGING

1. "Biography of John H. Glenn," NASA, November 12, 2008, accessed January 21, 2016, http://www.nasa.gov /centers/glenn/about/bios/glennbio.html.
2. "Thinking in Time: Theoretical and Methodological Issues in Aging Studies," Social Gerontology, accessed January 21, 2016, http://www.trinity.edu/mkearl/ger-time.html.
3. Progeria is a syndrome of unknown etiology that causes premature aging in children; it is also known as Hutchinson-Gilford syndrome. Affected children appear normal up to the first year of life. Gradually characteristics of the disorder become apparent—retarded growth and physical development, loss of body fat, absence of body hair, and baldness. Eventually the child develops dry, wrinkled skin, arteriosclerosis, and other conditions associated with old age. There is no treatment, and death occurs by the second decade.
4. "Thinking in Time: Theoretical and Methodological Issues in Aging Studies."
5. Jimmy Carter, *The Virtues of Aging* (New York: Ballantine, 1998), 10–11.
6. Ibid., 11.
7. "Administration on Aging (AoA): Income," Administration for Community Living, accessed January 15, 2016, http:// www.aoa.acl.gov/aging_statistics/profile/2014/9.aspx.
8. "Income and Poverty in the United States: 2013," US Census Bureau, September 2014, accessed January 21, 2016, https://www.census.gov/content/dam/Census /library/publications/2014/demo/p60-249.pdf.
9. "Administration on Aging (AoA): Housing," Administration for Community Living, accessed January 15, 2016, http://www.aoa.acl.gov/aging_statistics/profile/2014/11 .aspx.
10. Ibid.

11. "Administration on Aging (AoA): The Older Population," Administration for Community Living, accessed January 15, 2016, http://www.aoa.acl.gov/aging_statistics/profile /2014/3.aspx.

12. Ibid.

13. "Administration on Aging (AoA): Future Growth," Administration for Community Living, accessed January 15, 2016, http://www.aoa.acl.gov/aging_statistics /profile/2014/4.aspx.

14. "Administration on Aging (AoA): Living Arrangements," Administration for Community Living, accessed January 15, 2016, http://www.aoa.acl.gov/aging_statistics/profile /2014/6.aspx.

15. Ibid.

16. Ibid.

17. "Administration on Aging (AoA): Geographic Distribution," Administration for Community Living, accessed January 15, 2016, http://www.aoa.acl.gov/aging_statistics /profile/2014/8.aspx.

18. Ibid.

19. Benjamin Mandel and Livia Wu, "The Long and Short of Baby Boomer Balance Sheets: Multi-Asset Implications," J. P. Morgan Asset Management, October 2015, accessed January 21, 2016, https://am.jpmorgan.com/gi/getdoc /1383246462222.

20. Patricia Braus, "The Baby Boom at Mid-Decade," *American Demographics*, April 1995.

21. Ibid.

22. Ibid.

23. Carter, *Virtues of Aging*, 19.

24. Ibid.

25. Ibid., 20.

26. Linda Sage, "Senility Is Not a Normal Part of Aging, Study Suggests," Washington University School of Medicine in St. Louis, accessed 2000, http://news-info.wustl .edu/feature/1996/Apr96-Senility.

27. Mary Hager and Marc Peyser, "Lifestyle: Battling Alzheimer's," *Newsweek*, March 24, 1997.

28. Carter, *Virtues of Aging*, 51.
29. Ibid., 52.

CHAPTER 15
CROSSING THE BRIDGE

1. Taken from Acts 27:13–44.
2. Lawrence West, *Understanding Life*, 2d ed. (Freezone, AU: 1991, 1995), 6–7.
3. "Near-Death Experiences Illuminate Dying Itself," *New York Times*, October 28, 1986, accessed February 25, 2016, http://www.nytimes.com/1986/10/28/science/near-death-experiences-illuminate-dying-itself.html.
4. Current World Population, accessed February 25, 2016, http://www.worldometers.info/world-population.

APPENDIX A
HOW DIFFERENT NATIONS STACK UP

1. "Life Expectancy: Data by Country," Global Health Observatory, World Health Organization, accessed January 20, 2016, http://apps.who.int/gho/data/node.main.688.
2. "Austria: Statistics Summary (2002–Present)," Global Health Observatory, World Health Organization, accessed January 20, 2016, http://apps.who.int/gho/data/node.country.country-AUT.
3. "Life Expectancy: Data by Country."
4. "Finland: Statistics Summary (2002–Present)," Global Health Observatory, World Health Organization, accessed January 20, 2016, http://apps.who.int/gho/data/node.country.country-FIN?lang=en.
5. "Life Expectancy: Data by Country."
6. "Japan: Statistics Summary (2002–Present)," Global Health Observatory, World Health Organization, accessed January 20, 2016, http://apps.who.int/gho/data/node.country.country-JPN?lang=en.
7. "Life Expectancy: Data by Country."
8. "Switzerland: Statistics Summary (2002–Present)," Global Health Observatory, World Health Organization,

accessed January 20, 2016, http://apps.who.int/gho/data/node.country.country-CHE?lang=en.

9. "Life Expectancy: Data by Country."

10. "United States of America: Statistics Summary (2002–Present)," Global Health Observatory, World Health Organization, accessed January 20, 2016, http://apps.who.int/gho/data/node.country.country-USA?lang=en.

Appendix B
Average Life Expectancy of Males and Females in Four Developed Countries in 2013

1. "Life Expectancy: Data by Country."

CONNECT WITH US!

CHARISMA HOUSE

(Spiritual Growth)

 Facebook.com/CharismaHouse

 @CharismaHouse

Instagram.com/CharismaHouseBooks

SILOAM

(Health)

Pinterest.com/CharismaHouse

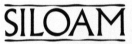

REALMS

(Fiction)

Facebook.com/RealmsFiction

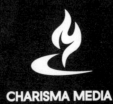